A PLUME BOOK

CANCER: 50 ESSENTIAL THINGS TO DO

GREG ANDERSON is the founder of the Cancer Recovery Foundation International group of charities, a global affiliation of national organizations whose mission is to help all people prevent and survive cancer.

Cancer Recovery Foundation focuses its work on developing and teaching integrated cancer care programs. The organization is a leading proponent of less-toxic and least-invasive cancer prevention and treatment research.

Greg Anderson was diagnosed with stage IV lung cancer in 1984. His surgeon gave him just thirty days to live. Refusing to accept the hopelessness of this prognosis, he went searching for people who had lived even though their doctors told them they were "terminal."

His findings from interviews with over 16,000 cancer survivors form the strategies and action points for what has become an international cancer recovery movement. Today, Anderson is widely recognized as one of the world's leading wellness authorities. He is the author of thirteen books, including the inspirational classic *The Cancer Conqueror*.

Make contact and find more information at www.cancer recovery.org.

D0095565

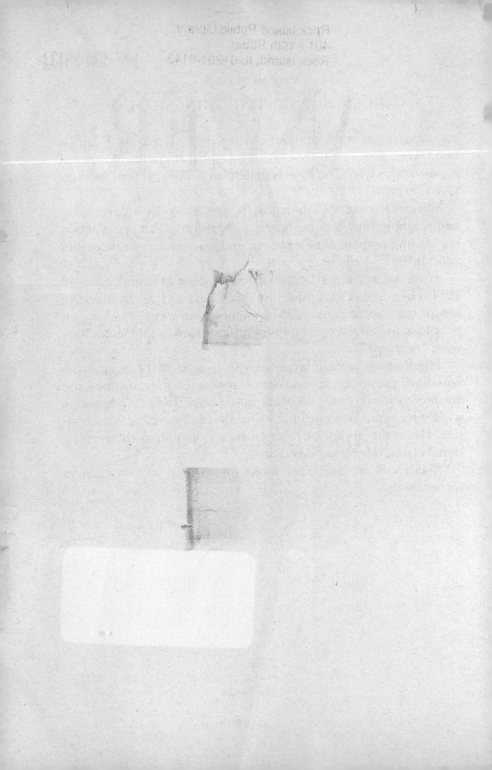

CANCER:

50 ESSENTIAL THINGS TO DO

2013 EDITION

GREG ANDERSON

A PLUME BOOK

PLUME
Published by the Penguin Group
Penguin Group (USA) Inc., 375 Hudson Street, New York, New York 10014, U.S.A. • Penguin Group
(Canada), 90 Eglinton Avenue East, Suite 700, Toronto, Ontario, Canada M4P 2Y3 (a division of Pearson
Penguin Canada Inc.) • Penguin Books Ltd., 80 Strand, London WC2R 0RL, England • Penguin Ireland,
25 St. Stephen's Green, Dublin 2, Ireland (a division of Penguin Books Ltd.) • Penguin Group (Australia),
707 Collins Street, Melbourne, Victoria 3008, Australia (a division of Pearson Australia Group Pty. Ltd.) •
Penguin Books India Pvt. Ltd., 11 Community Centre, Panchsheel Park, New Delhi – 110 017, India •
Penguin Group (NZ), 67 Apollo Drive, Rosedale, Auckland 0632, New Zealand (a division of Pearson New
Zealand Ltd.) • Penguin Books, Rosebank Office Park, 181 Jan Smuts Avenue, Parktown North 2193,
South Africa • Penguin China, B7 Jaiming Center, 27 East Third Ring Road North, Chaoyang District,
Beijing 100020, China

Penguin Books Ltd., Registered Offices: 80 Strand, London WC2R 0RL, England

First published by Plume, a member of Penguin Group (USA) Inc. An earlier edition of this book was
published by Plume under the title *50 Essential Things to Do When the Doctor Says It's Cancer.*

First Edition, March 1993
Second Edition, August 1999
Third Edition, March 2009
Fourth Edition, January 2013
10 9 8 7 6 5 4 3 2 1

Copyright © Greg Anderson, 1993, 1999, 2009, 2012
All rights reserved

Ⓟ REGISTERED TRADEMARK—MARCA REGISTRADA

LIBRARY OF CONGRESS CATALOGING-IN-PUBLICATION DATA

CIP data is available.
ISBN 978-0-452-29828-6

Printed in the United States of America

PUBLISHER'S NOTE
Every effort has been made to ensure that the information contained in this book is complete and accurate.
However, neither the publisher nor the author is engaged in rendering professional advice or services to
the individual reader. The ideas, procedures, and suggestions contained in this book are not intended
as a substitute for consulting with your physician. All matters regarding your health require medical
supervision. Neither the author nor the publisher shall be liable or responsible for any loss or damage
allegedly arising from any information or suggestion in this book.

While the author has made every effort to provide accurate telephone numbers, Internet addresses, and
other contact information at the time of publication, neither the publisher nor the author assumes any
responsibility for errors, or for changes that occur after publication. Further, publisher does not have any
control over and does not assume any responsibility for author or third-party Web sites or their content.

This book is dedicated to my wife, Linda.
Your unconditional loving sustains me.

CONTENTS

Part Two
The 50 Essential Things to Do

FOREWORD

In 1984, the same day my surgeon told me, "The tiger is out of the cage. Your lung cancer has come roaring back. I'd give you about thirty days to live," I turned to the work of O. Carl Simonton, M.D. Over the ensuing years, Carl became my teacher, mentor, colleague, and friend. His guidance literally saved my life.

In 2009, we both gave presentations at a conference in Heidelberg, Germany. At the end of my talk I presented Carl with Cancer Recovery Foundation's Lifetime Achievement Award. Every person in that huge auditorium rose and gave this giant of a man the longest, most thunderous standing ovation I have ever witnessed. The award and the audience response moved Carl to tears.

It was the last time I would see him alive. Carl died just a month later at his home in Malibu, California. He wrote the first foreword to this book. I now repeat it because it means so much to me.

From the Desk of O. Carl Simonton, M.D.

For over thirty-five years, I have been working with an approach to cancer that includes the physical, mental, and spiritual. I have treated thousands of patients with a relatively high rate of recovery, even from so-called terminal illness. I have learned a great deal about healing, and I have met some remarkable patients. Greg Anderson is one of them.

This book, *Cancer: 50 Essential Things to Do*, is a testimony to patients taking charge and choosing a stance of hope toward a diagnosis of cancer. Many of you who read this book are undoubtedly in a very difficult situation. Do not despair. Keep your hope alive. Learn from the experience of someone who was given a thirty-days-to-live prognosis. The author has been there. He knows what it's like to deal with the despair of cancer. He also knows what it's like to get well again.

While the road ahead may be difficult, I want you to know that it can be the most rewarding journey you will ever take. Even though the path through cancer requires work and discipline, it is also filled with discoveries that will excite and inspire you. Keep your focus on those joys.

Begin your journey now. Here, in this book, are the keys that can open the door for your return to good health. Take charge. Live this moment. Forgive. Love. You'll then know the power of hope . . . and you will be on the path to getting well again.

Simonton Cancer Center
Pacific Palisades, California

Simonton's work continues. You will find complete information at www.simontoncenter.com.

ACKNOWLEDGMENTS

A heartfelt thank-you to all the friends and colleagues of Cancer Recovery Foundation. I treasure you.

To all who so generously gave their time, talents, and creativity to this project, please accept my sincere appreciation.

And to all who search these pages for the answers to wellness, my encouragement and love.

INTRODUCTION

This revised and updated fourth edition of *Cancer: 50 Essential Things to Do* is written for those people who want to survive the experience of cancer and who are willing to actively participate in the recovery process. The book's goal is twofold: to help you gain a sense of clarity about the diagnosis you have been given, and to encourage you to design and implement an "integrated" cancer recovery plan that has your highest level of confidence.

"Integrated cancer care" is a term I introduced in the first edition of this book. It came out of the work my wife, Linda, and I started in early 1985. The previous year I was diagnosed with lung cancer—squamous cell carcinoma. I had my left lung removed. Four months later the cancer returned with a vengeance and was now metastatic to the ribs and lymph system—stage IV. Following a second surgery, I agreed to have radiation. I refused chemotherapy. My surgeon gave me thirty days to live.

From our kitchen table, I began a search for cancer survivors. Starting with referrals from other patients, I telephoned cancer patients everywhere. I would ask, "What did you do to get well and stay well?" I kept the focus on finding out "what went right" from the survivors; this, as opposed to orthodox medicine, which had all the focus on what was wrong.

The initial survivor interviews invariably led to discussions of dietary practices in addition to traditional medical care. Food was thought to be as important as medicine to many survivors. There were all sorts of nutritional theories. Some were quite odd, such as the "watermelon cure." But survivor after survivor emphasized a shift away from highly processed foods and toward "real" foods.

Many other survivors talked about the mind's role in healing. "Thinking positive" was a fundamental precept, as was having the will to live. Others spoke of the healing power of exercise, humor, purpose, play, sex, transpersonal psychology, and more.

Within a few months, we became a sort of clearinghouse for these ideas. Cancer patients and their families started calling us asking about "complementary and alternative medicine (CAM)," "merged therapies," "combination treatments," "linked protocols," and even "touch therapies." We produced a little four-page summary and sent it to all who asked. It was the humble beginnings of what today is a global outreach—Cancer Recovery Foundation International.

A survivor told us of the Preventive Medical Center of Marin. This was the first time I heard the description "integrative medicine." It struck a personal chord with me and we began to call our work "integrated cancer care." It was less than a year later that the esteemed Harvard-educated physician Andrew Weil, M.D., began to make integrative medicine a household word. Dr. Weil is to be credited with driving wide public interest in this subject, including professional interest at the academic medical level.

When Cancer Recovery Foundation uses the term "integrated," we mean patient-centered cancer care that extends well beyond the orthodox treatments of surgery, radiation, and chemotherapy. The fundamental focus of integrated cancer care is about displacing illness by creating wellness—physically, emotionally, and spiritually. Orthodox medicine often has a place, an important short-term role, in the cancer recovery process. But nutrition, exercise, and stress management, not medicine, form the basis of integrated cancer care. Also included are beliefs and attitudes, social support, creative thinking, and spirituality. Integrated cancer care requires patients to be active participants in their own health and healing. It views physicians as one of several possible health advisors, requiring those same health advisors to view patients as whole persons rather than simply a physical body or a disease. Finally, integrated cancer care is not to be confused with complementary and alternative treatment options. CAM options are techniques and protocols. Integrated cancer care is much more than that. For the vast majority of cancer patients who contact us, when we suggest integrated cancer care, we are actually suggesting a whole new way of life.

The Cancer Recovery Foundation, along with affiliated organizations, is today the world's leading proponent of integrated cancer care. Now nearly thirty years from humble beginnings, we are grateful to have dedicated staff in five countries and links with hundreds of health advisors around the globe. These include traditionally trained oncologists who honor and practice the tenets we teach. The guidance contained in this book is based on this vast knowledge base and experience.

This book is action-oriented, designed to help you the patient put in motion a program that will maximize your opportunity for a complete recovery while maintaining a high quality of life. This is not a book to be read and then put away, never to be referred to again. Instead, think of using this as your wellness resource guide for the next two years—a reasonable time for recovery. Return to it again and again to get "unstuck" in your cancer journey.

I believe this book has a meaningful message for every person touched by cancer. The strategies are tailor-made for the person with a recent cancer diagnosis. If you have been told "it's cancer," you'll find here the information you need to gain control over your fears, analyze your diagnosis, and put in place the most effective integrated cancer care program possible. For the newly diagnosed, I recommend following the "50 Essential Things" in order. There is a certain logical progression in their sequence.

Following this pattern will prove invaluable and will ensure that you are making the wisest decisions possible.

This book is also written for the person who has been diagnosed with a recurrence of cancer. Recurrence is a frightening event, a time of reevaluation medically, emotionally, and spiritually. I encourage you to make the "50 Essential Things" the very heart of your entire analysis. Thoughtfully follow the steps. Use this book as your primary guide. A recurrence does not equate with death. What you do does make a difference. See the "50 Essential Things" as mandatory points of action. Then you'll know you're doing everything possible to regain health.

THE WELLNESS AND RECOVERY JOURNAL

Before you begin your studies, secure a notebook and a pencil, or open a new folder on your laptop. I ask you to create a Wellness and Recovery Journal. I started mine with a single sheet of my daughter's notebook paper and an old three-ring binder. Nothing elaborate is required. As you read, questions and insights will come to mind. Write them down. You'll find yourself clipping newspaper and magazine articles about cancer. Put them in your notebook. This is going to become your primary source book, a reference manual for your personal and individual cancer recovery journey. Now, twenty-nine years after I was told I would die, I have a wealth of insights important to me. I still add information. My journal also serves as an excellent log of my cancer recovery journey.

I encourage you to do the same. You need the clarity the Wellness and Recovery Journal delivers. Even though a road map to recovery is contained in this book, each person must ultimately chart his or her own course to well-being. Use your Wellness and Recovery Journal to record your unique personal insights. Especially record your questions. Then ask. Ask your doctor, your medical technicians, and other survivors. Nothing is to be assumed. Ask about medical terms that you don't understand. Ask about reasons for tests. Ask about the results of those tests. Ask for success stories. Ask. Ask. Ask. Asking questions gives you significant power. Do not be intimidated by medical personnel, their processes, or their jargon. You are the one in charge. Ask! Then record the responses. Come back to them again and again.

Through it all, there is good reason to be filled with hope, provided you take an active part in the recovery process. Understand this recurring theme: You must not simply treat illness, you must also create wellness. It's integrated cancer care. It's your one best road to survival. Let's get started now.

Greg Anderson
The Woodlands, Texas
January 2013

AUTHOR'S NOTE

The ideas in this book are meant to supplement the care and guidance of competent medical professionals. At no time does the author suggest that these steps take the place of conventional medical treatment. Do not attempt a self-diagnosis. Do not embark upon self-treatment of a serious illness without professional help. There are a growing number of informed doctors who will work with their clients to integrate body, mind, and spirit. Find one. Form a healing partnership.

The characters in this book are composites of real people. They are not intended to portray specific individuals.

PART ONE

UNDERSTAND THE CANCER JOURNEY

THE EMERGING MODEL OF CANCER CARE

Healing requires a willingness to change—physically, emotionally, and spiritually.

The morning of December 31, 2005, I received a telephone call from Gretchen, a woman caught in the grip of uncontrolled panic. It was her husband, Robert. The previous afternoon, he received word that his head and neck cancer had spread. Despite state-of-the-art treatments at one of the world's leading cancer centers, treatment had failed. Now the doctors were insisting the only answer was removal of his right jawbone, a risky and difficult surgery that would likely result in permanent facial deformity and impaired speech. Even with the surgery, the outcome was uncertain at best.

The news was devastating to Robert. He openly spoke about committing suicide after hearing the news. Gretchen needed answers on how to help her husband—now.

Robert and I talked several times that day. He was a brilliant and articulate man with dual doctorate degrees who taught German at a prestigious private college in New Jersey. During his career, Robert was the recipient of numerous awards. His professional path seemed destined for even greater things. He was aware he was about to be nominated Dean of Students and Vice President of Academic Affairs, roles that gave him a very powerful voice in the school's administration. It was a goal he yearned for since his early days as an assistant professor in upstate New York. And now, his grim cancer diagnosis seemed to be blocking him from achieving that very goal.

Robert needed to talk, and I was there to listen. He shared about the difficulty of accepting the diagnosis of a malignant parotid gland. First, Robert felt the biopsy was botched. Following the pathology evaluation, the medical team recommended surgery, to be followed by radiation. But when Robert understood that a key facial nerve runs right through the parotid gland, he balked. It was common for this nerve to be damaged, even severed, during this complicated surgical procedure. It left many patients with impaired speech, the inability to control facial muscles, and even the loss of function of one's eyelid.

Robert openly railed against his surgeon's recommendations. He simply would not allow surgery. But he was open to a course of radiation therapy. And thus his cancer treatment began.

Throughout his life, Robert had limited interest in diet or exercise. However, after this initial diagnosis, he learned everything he could about cancer and nutrition. He became a vegan and lost nearly thirty pounds, which helped lower his high blood pressure. And for the first time in his life, he began to exercise—a thirty-minute daily walk, rain or shine. As Robert put it, "For the first time in my life I began telling my body to be well." During my first conversation with Robert after Gretchen's worried phone call, I praised him on the changes he made to help bring his body to a place of greater wellness. Still, he was dismissive of my compliments and encouragements on his new diet and exercise regimen. As we ended the first call, Robert remained despondent.

Near the end of a second call that December day, I brought up the issue of Robert's emotions after hearing the news. Robert was angry—with his diagnosis, with his doctors, and with his own body. Raising his voice, he called one of his oncologists "an idiot" and "intellectually dishonest" because she recommended chemotherapy even though these treatments have little proven success. But Robert was angry not just about his cancer diagnosis and prognosis, he was also angry about life. His tone of voice was critical and confrontational, and his statements were sprinkled with profanities. I felt as if my every word was being challenged.

Earlier in the day, Gretchen shared that they reached me through the phone numbers in one of my books. I asked Robert to read the chapter entitled "Choose Your Emotional Style." My suggestion was not well received and he abruptly ended the call.

Within an hour, Gretchen was back on the phone. Robert wanted to talk. This time he started with the question, "Why do you believe there is a God?" His inquiry started a fascinating discussion.

Before his diagnosis, Robert had no time for or interest in spirituality. "I haven't had anything positive to say about religion for over forty years," he mused. But then he shared that one night, just as he was drifting off to sleep, he clearly heard a voice that said, *Follow me*. Robert continued almost reverently, "There is no mistaking that the voice was very real and very close. The tone of the voice was gentle and loving. And as I thought about the encounter later, all I could think of was, 'Follow whom?' and 'Who is this?'"

Since that time, Robert could not get the voice off his mind. After thinking about the command for several weeks, he stopped at a church that he often passed on his daily walk. Upon entering he lit one of the votive candles in the rack near the back of the sanctuary. Then he knelt in a pew and was quiet. Looking at the main altar, Robert observed a beautiful golden piece of art depicting Jesus hanging on a cross.

Of course, Robert had seen this image many times before. Previously he either ignored or scoffed at it. Now, in a quiet and reverent tone of voice, Robert shared how he stared, transfixed at the crucifix for what may have been thirty minutes or more. Finally he spoke out loud: "Was that you saying 'Follow me'?"

"I left that church more hopeful than I had been in months," Robert shared. "And to this day I continue to explore what truth there may be in a spiritual quest."

Later, I pondered Robert's experience. It was similar to those I have seen and heard in literally thousands of cancer survivors. The quest is not necessarily a religious transformation. Clearly for Robert it was not, as he still struggles with the idea of a Divine Force. Rather, the difference can be understood as being based in hope. More specifically, in a conscious decision to replace despair and helplessness with hope and trust that all will be well no matter what the outcome. Hope is a subject we will have a great deal to say about throughout this book.

My sense is that I left Robert more settled that day. The anger and hostility were gone from his voice. He was obviously calmer and seemed more at peace. And he was understanding more how his diet and exercise routines could significantly contribute to his recovery.

Robert did not attempt to end his life that New Year's Eve. I like to think I had some part in that. He eventually went ahead with the recommended surgery, refused chemotherapy, and within two years was declared cancer-free, much to the surprise of his medical oncologist. About two years ago, I met Robert and Gretchen for the first time. While Robert does not have impaired speech, he does have a noticeable facial deformity. "But he grew this nice beard," said a smiling Gretchen as she playfully tugged at his thick gray Santa-style growth. "Nobody knows."

Robert and I keep in touch. "I still don't know about God," he says, "but I have come to a point in my life of knowing a deep peace. And I am becoming increasingly thankful for the smallest of graces—the sight of a sunrise, the fragrance of a flower, and the touch of my wife's hand. I've been able to see things more clearly and hardly ever get angry at the small stuff." In a holiday card, he said that, symbolically, he believes that the reason his cancer was found in his neck was so that his words would be softer and he could become more compassionate.

I kept Robert's holiday card. It's a perfect thumbnail of the integrated cancer care journey. Medicine? Yes, in careful, less-toxic, least-invasive doses. Excellent nutrition? Of course. Robert opted to go the vegan route. Exercise? Daily. Emotional intelligence? Robert is becoming increasingly skilled at releasing hostility. Spirituality? He is more peaceful, grateful, and hopeful than at any time in his life.

THE TUMOR MODEL

Robert's embrace of a holistic integrated cancer care program offers a powerful alternative to the current orthodox cancer treatment paradigm so widely practiced by oncologists and accepted, without serious questioning, by cancer patients. The fact is that current conventional Western cancer treatment is exclusively focused on the disease—the tumor model. Following a myriad of tests, a diagnosis is made. Once diagnosed, the tumor or the blood-based cancer is attacked with surgery, chemotherapy, and/or radiation. Medical expertise is required to prescribe and administer these treatments, and thus a different specialist is present to implement each treatment modality. The entire process is focused on the tumor, and precious little about the person.

One person whom Cancer Recovery Foundation helped evaluate the spectrum of treatment options was a medical doctor, a family practitioner named Ruth. She was two years into treatment for a stage II infiltrating ductal carcinoma—an early-stage breast cancer. Things were not going well. Her experience started with the way she was treated as a person. Prior to her initial surgery, she was told she needed a CT scan to determine if the tumor had attached to the chest wall. Ruth knew CT scans were not routinely used in a stage II breast cancer diagnosis, but the surgeon was insistent, saying he needed to know whether or not the tumor could be removed with mastectomy. Ruth's discomfort with the test was summarily dismissed, and reluctantly, she agreed.

The test did not go well. CT scans, also called CAT scans or computerized tomography scans, require a dye, a contrast solution, to be injected into your arm through an intravenous line prior to the test. I recall Ruth's anger as she shared her experiences with me. "The technician who tried to insert the IV didn't know what the hell he was doing. First, he couldn't find a vein. Then he dropped the entire IV kit on the floor. Instead of throwing it away and requesting a sterile one, he picked it up and was about to use this germ-laden apparatus on me. I yelled at him, 'Stop it!' And I walked out the door."

"He didn't know who I was," continued Ruth. "He cared only about the procedure and nothing about me, his patient. I sat in that god-awful gown in that cold exam room and was afforded no human comfort, no respect, and no acknowledgment that I was a living and breathing human being, let alone a medical professional. It was all about the cancer. At that moment, I had this sinking feeling. I realized the system in which I was trained, and in which I practiced, would eventually fail me."

Unfortunately, Ruth's experience is far from unusual. The tumor model of cancer treatment is often coldly and cruelly dispassionate—the patient a secondary thought to the disease. In Cancer Recovery Foundation's work, cancer patients most often turn to us after the system has in some way failed them. Some patients are concerned about the tests used to arrive at their diagnosis. Others feel as if they are being rushed, even forced, into treatments without understanding their options. Many cancer patients reach out to us only after traditional medical treatments have failed and they are told the frightening words, "Your cancer is back." It is often at these points of systemic failure that our phone rings.

THE SHIFT

Since the focus of the tumor-based model is solely on the tumor, little if any effort is expended in exploring the benefits of healthful diet, regular exercise, immune-enhancing treatments, social and emotional support, spirituality, or other methods to enhance a patient's well-being. And as so often happens, a focus solely on the tumor leaves the thinking patient disempowered and unable to contribute to their own healing. In fact, empowering cancer patients and their support team may be one of the most important aspects of our work. If Cancer Recovery Foundation can equip you, along with tens of thousands of additional cancer patients, to fully understand and practice integrated cancer care, we will have changed the singular treatment mind-set in cancer.

Let's be clear: surgery, chemotherapy, and radiation can play an important role in cancer treatment. But with most cancers, especially early-stage cancer, the benefits conventional treatment may provide must be carefully weighed against the risks.

Conventional treatments do not address the underlying factors that predispose one to, or prevent, cancer development. Conventional cancer treatments merely treat *symptoms*. The tumor model of cancer considers the tumor the entire problem and ignores factors like tobacco use and obesity that directly affect the development of lung, breast, prostate, and colorectal cancers. The orthodox approach says, in essence, "See, there's the tumor. That's the problem. That's what we will attack."

Converse to this narrowly defined approach, the emerging model of cancer treatment recognizes the tumor as a physical indication of a greater underlying imbalance. The new model of cancer care recognizes the growing evidence that shows that supporting and creating high levels of well-being with nutrition and exercise is at least as important as conventional cancer treatment. In addition to the nutrition and exercise emphasis, the broader aspects of emotional, social, and spiritual support from this model of treatment can be critically important to optimal health—so critical as to create a level of well-being that transcends disease. The multipronged approach of integrated cancer care and treatment recognizes the importance of the person as a whole, rather than just the cancer. It is a critical distinction. Please grasp the importance of this truth in your own journey: your cancer is not just about the tumor.

Science is beginning to discover what ancient healers from a variety of cultures and disciplines have known and practiced for centuries—that our mind and body and spirit are inseparable. Together they create a "life force" that nurtures health, healing, and the optimal functioning of our immune system. This means that health is much more than healthcare, and that cancer care is much more than cancer treatment.

Understanding and acknowledging that our body and mind and spirit are inseparable, the emerging paradigm of cancer care provides optimal support for the whole person. These disciplines can be naturally and safely integrated with conventional cancer treatments if the patient desires. Supporting overall health and well-being supports immune function, which facilitates the healing process, improves our quality of life, and enhances recovery. In short, the wise integration of body, mind, and spirit helps create health and encourages healing.

The study of the relationship between the mind, body, and immune system is called psychoneuroimmunology. Scientists are discovering that when we feel empowered, our immune system is empowered. Fear can have a substantial negative impact on immune function, whereas regaining a sense of control and positive engagement in our own health and healing helps support immune function. The principles of empowerment, self-engagement, and personal choice are at the heart of the emerging model of cancer care.

More than any other dynamic, the emerging model understands that mind, body, spirit, and immune system are one. Moving away from the single-dimension tumor model of cancer, we are progressing toward multiple ways of supporting mind, body, spirit, and immune function that include exercise, nutrition, stress reduction, and spirituality. Like our professor friend Robert found, all are interrelated, contributing to the benefit provided by the others in a synergistic way. By engaging in the many ways we can support mind, body, and spirit, we clearly optimize our body's healing potential. Today, we can say with certainty that a cancer recovery program without integration of body, mind, and spirit is an incomplete program at best.

Thousands of cases of recovery from "incurable" life-threatening diseases, including advanced cancers, have been scientifically documented. I am one of those documented cases. There is no question you also possess that potential.

While research of this phenomenon is still in its infancy, a growing cadre of physicians, practitioners, and allied healthcare professionals are coming forward to serve cancer patients in optimally engaging in their own health and healing. With growing scientific interest in this field, researchers have begun to study patients who have recovered from seemingly impossible circumstances in hopes of beginning to understand how we all can better facilitate our body's remarkable healing abilities. I am asking you to act now to design and implement your own integrated cancer recovery program. In fact, if you are dealing with a diagnosis of cancer, there has never been a better time or more important time to fully embrace this program.

THE QUESTION OF CAUSE

In our work, we have found a marked propensity for patients to ask, "What caused my cancer?" It is an understandable question. In my own case, I had to look no further than cigarettes to find an immediate answer. But as I researched further, the cause of my lung cancer was more than just smoking. At the time of my diagnosis, I was overwhelmed by the pressures of a new baby, a cross-country move, a new job, a fast-food diet, and a feeling that I was inadequate as a husband, father, and professional. Now, twenty-nine years later, it is clear this combination of factors, not just the tobacco, was the cause of my lung cancer.

There is no one cause for all cancers. If you or a loved one are dealing with cancer and wrestling with the cause question, examine your personal terrain—physically, emotionally, and even spiritually. You will likely find many factors contributed to your cancer development. These include diet, exercise, toxin exposure, vitamin D levels, hormones, certain medical tests, and even some medical treatments, as well as factors that can't necessarily be controlled, like gender, age, genetics, race, and emotional makeup. These factors, interacting together, impact cancer development. For each person, the combination will be different. The emerging model of care recognizes this complexity.

On the cellular level, cancer is an expression of genes that have mutated, resulting in cells that have gone awry. But bad inherited genes are not the cause of 90 to 95 percent of cancers. An unlucky draw from the genetic pool explains just 5 to 10 percent of the causal factors.

Genes gone badly are more often the outcome of many other factors. Your genes turn "off" and "on" in relation to the environmental factors in which those genes live. The good news is that even if we do have a gene that potentially predisposes us to cancer, lifestyle factors can and will impact the degree to which that gene is expressed.

Dr. Dean Ornish, one of the world's most esteemed pioneers and integrated healthcare revolutionaries stated, "People should realize that genes may be our predisposition, but they are not our fate. The fact is massive positive changes in genetic activity are generated through lifestyle choices. Our choices are as powerful as our strongest drugs and occur rapidly in most individuals."

How powerful? Among the researchers who study lifestyle's impact on health, there is a consensus that 50 to 75 percent of cancers are totally and completely preventable. Breast cancer is the most common cancer diagnosis among women and prostate cancer the most common for men. Excellent and compelling scientific evidence exists today that shows eight out of ten breast cancers could be prevented—stopped before a diagnosis was even made. Science demonstrating similar promising results for prostate cancer is emerging, proving that cancer does not have to be as black and white as once thought.

These developments are startling revelations to the idea of prevention in its effectiveness to ward off cancer. Prevention is accomplished by minimizing or eliminating factors that predispose one to cancer development. As we'll discuss in greater depth later in this book, reducing the consumption of sugar and animal fats, avoiding inactivity, eliminating the use of tobacco, moderating the consumption of alcohol, and adding nutritional supplements that reduce genetic expression are all excellent preventative measures.

If you have been recently diagnosed, you may be asking, "So how does this help me? I already have cancer." The good news is that many of these same steps can also contribute to your getting well and staying well. If many cancers can be prevented through lifestyle measures, common sense tells us that these same healthful self-care measures will also be of value in both the recovery process and in reducing the risk of recurrence. Happily, there is a significant and growing body of research that supports the huge role that self-care plays in cancer treatment.

Think back for a moment to Robert, our professor friend. He made shifts in his diet, his exercise, and his emotional disposition, and he even had a spiritual encounter that left him a changed man. These self-care factors, combined with his medical treatment, have resulted in a positive outcome. It is a pattern we have observed literally thousands of times in our work at Cancer Recovery Foundation.

There exists significant resistance to these "natural healing" ideas in much of the conventional orthodox oncology community. Even though Hippocrates, the father of modern medicine, said over 2,500 years ago, "Let food be thy medicine and thy medicine thy food," many Western-trained oncologists have little tolerance for such ideas. Both my surgeon and radiation oncologist told me to eat whatever I wanted when I was undergoing radiation therapy. They were more concerned that I ate anything, sugars and fats included, in order to maintain weight, than the quality of what I was putting in my body. If there were ever a time to stop drinking soda and eating candy and give up French fries, cancer is it. We will cover much more in the way of specific dietary suggestions in a later section of this book.

Like most of us, doctors are busy people. Most do their very best to keep apprised of everything that is going on in their field.

The good ones constantly read new scientific studies published in professional journals, attend conferences, and see pharmaceutical representatives several times a year. But as a result of their own immersion in the field, there is a pervasive assumption that "If it were true, I would know about it." Nutrition and the more natural self-care approaches are often dismissed, despite the mounting body of evidence that points to their significance.

Nutrition, exercise, social support, and mind/body and spiritual matters are barely, if ever, on the curriculum in medical school. Following a talk I gave at the world-famous M.D. Anderson Cancer Center in Houston, Texas, a medical oncologist pulled me aside and said, "My patients don't want to change what they eat. And they sure don't want to exercise. They want their treatment and then they want to forget about cancer."

My response is that patients should do all possible to help prevent and control cancer in ways that do not harm the body. Others have lamented that there are no "double blind studies" to prove that these facets of emerging healthcare—changes to diet, exercise, and thought—are not harmful to the patient. This is demonstrative of the medical cultural bias that dismisses natural self-help approaches in favor of pharmaceutical solutions. The demand for "hard science" stands in the way of common sense.

Of course it is important to note that people who exercise regularly and eat healthfully can still develop cancer. Clearly, cancer is not a single-cause disease. And for each person the combination of causative factors is different. However, we can all learn to take better care of ourselves physically, emotionally, and spiritually. A diagnosis of cancer is the signal to do so, providing an opportunity to fully love and care for oneself. That truth stands as the premier attribute of the emerging model of cancer care.

BEYOND THE CAUSE: YOUR RESPONSE

After nearly thirty years of guiding cancer patients, this much I know for certain: the patients who do well actively participate in creating health and enhancing their well-being. When we engage in our own process of recovery, we regain a sense of autonomy, a feeling of control that we can impact our own health and life, a sense of being in charge. Numerous studies have shown that patients who become actively involved in designing their recovery plan are more likely to follow through with their treatments, less likely to have complications, and more likely to have favorable outcomes than those who simply take a passive role.

I do realize that becoming an active patient has its own challenges. Being told that you have cancer is a very frightening experience. Due to the technical nature of conventional cancer treatments, those decisions tend to be driven by specialists. At this point, patients often become passive bystanders in their own care. Overwhelmed by procedures, treatments, and side effects that they may not understand, they often acquiesce without understanding their options.

There are also haunting questions in the minds of most cancer patients about their pre-diagnosis role. I often hear statements like, "Why me? What did I do wrong? What could I have done differently? Am I to blame for my cancer?" These questions are a natural response to a life-threatening diagnosis. While natural, they can generate thoughts and feelings of worry, despair, self-blame, and even resentment toward others. Misunderstanding one's role very often adds further stress to an already challenging situation.

As a consequence, cancer patients are often left feeling isolated, frightened, and depressed, a state that inhibits both immune function and healing. In this context, patients may be left feeling unable to contribute in a meaningful way to their recovery and, as a result, feel a sense of loss of control over their own health.

In Cancer Recovery Foundation's work, we help patients reframe their experience away from possible blame, self-recrimination, or disempowering fear. Instead, we assist them in gaining a broader understanding of cancer and the healing process, help them to develop self-compassion, and support them in creating a practical action plan. In this way patients develop a sense of regaining control and being in charge of their lives and health. And that sense of control is a central element that helps in one's healing.

Whether you are active or passive, you have a major influence on your own healing, positive or negative. Respected psychiatrist and cancer researcher Dr. David Spiegel wrote, "Medicine has focused so much on attacking the tumor that it has tended to ignore the body coping with the tumor, and the social and psychological variables that influence the somatic response to tumor invasion. Biologic treatments that produce only marginal increases in survival are widely employed despite considerable risks and side effects. Many psychosocial practices such as support groups, mind/body practices and simple relaxation that are clearly helpful and carry with them very little in the way of risks, side effects, or expense, are far less widely employed."

When we engage in creating our own health and healing within a broader holistic context, we become an active and inspired participant in optimally supporting our mind, body, spirit, and immune system. Reclaiming a sense of being in charge of our own life and health is a vitally important foundation of the healing process. By doing so, our immune system is enhanced and we begin to actively work toward creating our own foundations for healing and recovery.

Personal autonomy, personal choice, and the right to choose one's own treatments are important foundations of integrated cancer care. All of the complementary medical therapies we will discuss in this book are designed to support health and build immune function. And they are meant to do so in the least toxic and most minimally invasive manner.

Yet for many cancer patients, nutrition and exercise seem to lack the same scientific basis accorded surgery, radiation, or chemotherapy. And it's true. For some of these complementary therapies, there is substantial scientific evidence that supports their use. For others, less research exists. I recognize that scientific evidence is a very helpful guide to choosing treatments. Evidence-informed care is valuable. But as Einstein said, "Not everything that counts can be counted and not everything that can be counted, counts." Trusting your own wisdom is also an exceedingly helpful guide to choosing treatments. My goal in this book is to guide you to merge science with your inner wisdom to make choices that are optimal for you.

The shift to the new model in health honors both the contribution and the limitations of orthodox cancer care. Let's be clear. By removing or killing tumor cells, conventional cancer treatments can play a valuable role in reducing the tumor load with which the body has to deal. However, since many conventional cancer treatments also have negative effects on healthy cells, these same treatments are often associated with significant side effects that can substantially reduce both immune function and quality of life. Even worse, the long-term negative health consequences of these treatments often mean compromised health for the rest of one's life.

More natural therapies function in an entirely different way. The goal of these therapies is to support the immune system and health and thus facilitate the body's own healing abilities. They work together with the body to promote healing. Through this synergistic action, complementary therapies can support the body's health and improve quality of life. Side effects from complementary treatment therapies are far less common.

Not one of the nearly 10,000 people who have participated in our cancer recovery program has ever developed a serious side effect from any of the complementary cancer therapies we have suggested. Hippocrates is also credited with instructing his students, "Above all, do no harm," and "Honor the healing power of Nature." These principles guide the recommendations you will read in this book.

The vast majority of participants in our program employ both conventional protocols and integrated modalities in combination. We help participants understand and choose those therapies that are right for them. This results in a truly individualized integrated cancer care program. By providing information, choices, and options, personal autonomy is enhanced and healing is better facilitated.

Remember, *you* have the central role. Your response to a cancer diagnosis is critical. The shift to the new model of care recognizes the growing evidence that supporting and creating high levels of well-being with nutrition, exercise, stress management, and emotional awareness is as important as any conventional cancer treatment. And the broader aspects of social and spiritual support can be critically important to optimal health so as to create a level of well-being that simply transcends disease, even a diagnosis of life-threatening cancer. The new model of care is grounded in igniting your natural ability to get well and stay well. Your role is to engage the whole you by creating health and well-being physically, emotionally, and even spiritually.

Cancer is not entirely about the tumor or the treatment. It's about you. And if you will respond, that is very good news indeed.

THE TRUE
SOURCES OF
HEALTH AND
HEALING

The central reason for writing this book is to help people with cancer understand the pivotal role they can choose to play in their own healing and eventual recovery. But in the minds of millions of people, a diagnosis of cancer means there is little room for anyone other than a team of specialists, doctors, and healthcare providers who will hopefully fix the problem. This belief is wrong, very wrong.

Yes, cancer patients need competent medical guidance and assistance. But all the medical treatment in the world will not and cannot create health and result in healing. Health is much more than healthcare. And it is important for those cancer patients who wish to survive and even thrive to take personal responsibility for doing all they can to get well and stay well—to find health and nurture true healing.

Where do we find health? How can we know healing? For the cancer patient, these are foundational questions. Thankfully, there is a hierarchy of answers.

THE WILL TO LIVE

The will to live, a psychological force found within all of us, is your starting point. It can be easily understood as the *inner desire for survival.* The will to live is the most basic requirement for the cancer journey.

Like all creatures, human beings have a fierce instinct for survival. Sometimes the biology of cancer will dictate the course of events regardless of the patient's attitude and fighting spirit. These events are often beyond our control. But patients with a positive attitude are clearly better able to cope with disease-related problems.

I have had hundreds of conversations with physicians who often observe how two patients of similar ages, with the same diagnosis, sharing a similar degree of illness and virtually identical treatment programs, experience vastly different outcomes. One of the few apparent differences was that one patient was pessimistic and the other optimistic. We have known for over 2,000 years, from the writings of Plato and Galen, that there is a direct correlation between the mind, the body, and one's health. "The cure of many diseases is unknown to physicians," Plato concluded, "because they are ignorant of the whole. For the part can never be well unless the whole is well."

The new emerging model of cancer care recognizes that the psychological and the physical elements of a body are not separate, isolated, and unrelated. Health is increasingly recognized as a balance of many factors, including physical and environmental elements, emotional and psychological states, nutritional and exercise habits, and more.

The will to live can be accurately seen as the starting point of health and healing. Believe it. Your will to live plays a large role in your recovery. The mind's role in causing and curing disease has been endlessly debated. No studies have proven in a scientifically valid way that a person can control the course of his or her cancer with the mind alone. However, there are millions of individuals who attest to the power of positive attitude and emotions.

I am one of those individuals. I purposely cultivated and strengthened my will to live. You can, too.

I often ask survivors to explain how they were able to transcend their health challenges. However diverse they are in ethnic or cultural background, age, gender, educational level, or type of illness, they have all gone through a similar process of a psychological shift. Virtually all consciously made a *decision to live*. After an initial period of feeling devastated, they simply decided to assess their new reality and live—however long that may be.

In my own case, the decision to live meant that I wanted to enjoy life and get more out of it, and most important, to believe that a cancer diagnosis did not mean my life was over. It also meant that I was willing to do whatever was needed to make the very most of each day.

The threat of death often renews our appreciation of the importance of life, love, friendship, and all there is to enjoy. We open up to new possibilities and begin taking risks we didn't have the courage to take before. Many patients have told me that facing the uncertainties of living with an illness makes life more meaningful. The smallest pleasures are intensified and much of the hypocrisy in life is eliminated. When pettiness, bitterness, and anger begin to dissipate, there is still a capacity for joy. I want that for you.

Hope: The Force That Sets Your Course

Combining the will to live with hope creates health and healing on many levels.

Cicero, the Roman statesman, is credited with the phrase, "While there is life, there is hope." I believe those words have greater power in reverse: "While there is hope, there is life." Hope comes first, life follows. Hope is the force that sets your course, inspiring the will to live and generating healing on every level.

The dictionary defines hope as *a feeling that what is wanted can be had, that events will turn out for the best.* That definition is not strong enough. Hope can best be defined as a *deeply confident expectation.* It is a force, a mental, emotional, and spiritual power, a strength you possess. Hope gives power to life to continue, expand, reach out, and go on. Hope is the miracle medicine of the mind. It inspires the will to live. Hope is the patient's greatest ally.

I ask that you stop to consider the importance of hope in your cancer journey. Please allow me to gently, lovingly ask you three questions:

Do you carry a vision of yourself as struggling or victorious?
Do you believe crippling disease or vibrant health is in your future?
Do you live most of each day filled with helplessness or infused with hopefulness?

How you envision yourself and perceive your circumstances has a great deal to do with your actual life experience. It's true in all areas of life—our relationships, our work, and especially our health.

One essential key to unlocking health is to carry a vision of hope. Hope revives ideals, renews dreams, and revitalizes visions. It scales the peak, wrestles with the impossible, and achieves the highest aim. Carry this truth deep in your heart: as long as you have hope, you are not helpless and no situation is hopeless.

A powerful act in creating health and healing is to choose the words you speak. Our words sometimes may spring forth without thought. But we have a choice in what we say. We can stop speaking about our problems and start speaking of our healing. The more we speak of solutions, as if they already exist, the less powerful our problems become. I ask that from this moment forward you begin to speak only of health and of healing. When you do, you plant the seeds to help create that reality.

A surgeon once admonished me, "You're spreading false hope." My response was, "I believe there is no such thing as false hope.

I believe there is only reasonable hope." However, in the world of cancer, there is a great deal of *false no-hope*. In medicine, that often takes the form of words like, "There's nothing more we can do." Or, "You have only a few months to live." Don't believe it.

Clearly, it is unrealistic to pretend that nothing bad ever happens to us. Bad things do happen to good people. Cancer is one of those bad things. Pretending otherwise is not the answer. Nor is playing word games to make ourselves sound psychologically strong or spiritually pure. When bad things happen, admit it. Acknowledge the cancer, but keep your thoughts focused on the most hopeful outcome.

We simply must take personal responsibility for our thoughts and words. As long as we keep making excuses and blame our family tree, our doctor, or a higher power, we will never be truly well.

I say this gently and lovingly: it's not the diagnosis of cancer that has you struggling and depressed. No. It's your thoughts about your diagnosis and circumstances that keep you down.

In front of the Cancer Recovery Group's offices is a 5,000-pound slab of Vermont granite. On it I had inscribed "Hope Rock," and then added two essential rules. Here they are:

Rule 1: There is always hope.
Rule 2: If someone says there is no hope, re-read rule 1.

Believe it. There is always hope. Let that sink deep into your mind and spirit. Hope is the force that sets your course. Follow the rules. Set your compass on hope. Keep your mind filled with victory! It is one of the great sources of health and healing.

SPIRITUAL CONNECTION: INNER GUIDANCE

Healing is a very personal journey, unique for each of us. At our deepest intuitive levels, most of us know many of the important things we need to do to get well and stay well. However, millions of us have forgotten how to listen to and trust our intuitive inner wisdom. Connecting with your own sense of what it means to be spiritual is an essential ingredient in defining your path to wellness.

I have come to understand that cancer is a call to listen to your Self—your Inner Healer, your deeper wisdom. Caught up in life's busyness, we often forget how to relax the mind and quiet the spirit. But it is only when we can be at peace and surrender to our deeper wisdom that we can receive the inner guidance so essential to healing.

I ask you to begin today to quiet your mind long enough to discover your own healing pathway. What you will find is both surprising and exciting. Research in psychospiritual reality confirms what healers and spiritual teachers have known for centuries—at the level of Self, we are far more aware and knowledgeable than at the level of our conscious mind.

Prayer is one method of rediscovering our Self. For some people, this spiritual journey may be expressed through a religious framework. For others, spirituality is expressed through a connection with Nature or a similar quest. The common thread is to connect with our deepest authentic Self. And for the skeptics, we now even have early research to show that this quest can activate the immune system, promote healing, and increase the possibilities for recovery.

In our work, we have found the spiritual journey to healing can be reliably and predictably started with three practices—forgiveness, gratitude, and unconditional love.

Forgiveness is our letting go of hurts and grievances. To be clear, it is our offering of forgiveness to others, not our receipt of forgiveness from others, which makes the difference. Most of us know at a deep level the thoughts of recrimination and remorse to which we cling. It was only after I forgave my father that I was able to reclaim health and receive the gift of healing. Release. Let go. Forgive.

Gratitude is a state of living and being that is consciously aware of and appreciative of the countless blessings and kindnesses we receive each and every moment. So very often on the cancer journey, our sense of gratitude can be clouded, momentarily obscured by helplessness, doubt, and despair. But when we observe and affirm the good things in life, we see them set aside these negative thoughts.

Unconditional loving—I like the word *loving* rather than the word *love*, as it better communicates the action required to make love real—is the essential practice of spiritual connection. Unconditional loving is another and higher state of Self. It comprises a giving, a creative flow, and a harmony. It's the acceptance of the human condition as perfectly imperfect. And it is a choice to love without any conditions; no "ifs" are allowed.

Forgiveness, gratitude, and unconditional loving. They are the gateway to your Self, to spiritual connection and inner guidance—one of the most powerful sources of health and healing. We will have more to say on these in the "50 Essential Things to Do."

RELATIONSHIPS: EMOTIONAL INTELLIGENCE AND SUPPORT

One of the great wellsprings of healing is an intimate group of supportive friends. When combined with a keen understanding of our own emotional makeup, the environment for healing is optimized.

Fear, anger, guilt. Happiness, contentment, love: they are all part of the roller coaster of human experience. Emotions are especially vivid when we are dealing with a life-threatening illness. In the cancer experience we cannot expect to prevent negative emotions altogether, nor should we expect to experience positive feelings every moment. But what we can do is acknowledge our feelings and refuse to get stuck in the negative ones. That often takes the help of one or more true friends.

You and I have the power to choose our emotions. Recall the concept that body, mind, and spirit all work together. Emotions are clearly part of that mix. When we recognize that our every thought, word, and behavior affects our greater health and well-being, we have then begun to learn the language of emotions.

Please understand that your emotions actually do manifest in your physical body and yield physical sensations. Take anxiety as an example. You may be anxious over an upcoming series of medical tests. Before long, you notice you have an upset stomach. Your first response might be to avoid or deny the connection. But if we stop and become aware of the sequence of thoughts and emotions, we link them to our bodily reactions. As a result, we can respond in a more intelligent way.

With practice, we can become skilled at identifying and observing our emotions. Once we can put words to the emotions— "That's fear that I am feeling," for example, we tend to resist the urge to fight the emotion. Instead, we can allow the emotion to work through without repression or strong reaction. As a result, we begin to experience more ease, more joy, and more spontaneity in our lives. We are able to claim a more honest relationship with ourselves. As a result, our relationships with others also become more authentic.

Research in the field of psychoneuroimmunology attests to the central role emotions play in the healing process. Landmark studies have demonstrated that simply meeting with others once a week to share emotionally and provide mutual support improves one's sense of well-being and significantly improves the chance of recovery from life-threatening illness. UCLA psychiatrist and cancer researcher Dr. Fawzy I. Fawzy found that malignant melanoma cancer patients randomly assigned to participate in a weekly support group for a six-week period after diagnosis showed an increased survival threefold over a five-year period compared to the control group. Six months after the group sessions ended, two-thirds of the patients in the support groups showed an increase of 25 percent or more in what are called natural killer cells, cancer-fighting cells in the immune system. No such increase was found in the control group.

In San Francisco, Dr. David Spiegel found women with metastatic breast cancer who attended a weekly support meeting lived on average twice as long as those who did not. Patients were encouraged to express their feelings about the illness and its effect on their lives. Spiegel found that the emotional repression and social isolation so often found among breast cancer patients was countered by participation in these groups. Importantly, he also noted that group members encouraged one another to be more assertive with their doctors.

In Arizona, Dr. Karen Weihs demonstrated that for women diagnosed with breast cancer, a large group of supportive friends and relatives is associated with a 60 percent reduction in recurrence and death compared to women with breast cancer who were socially isolated.

It's clear. Emotional connection with one's family and friends and emotional awareness of one's self plays a pivotal role in the healing process. As you spend time with those you love, do not simply rehearse the problems of cancer. Instead, share with these people how important they are in your life. And recognize that the contribution made by their support is as important as any cancer therapy.

MIND/BODY: VISUALIZING THE DESIRED OUTCOME

I will emphasize this once again: you possess incredible healing potential. For many people, the body's ability to heal remains a greatly underutilized resource. In large part, it is because many people have forgotten how to listen to the healing messages our bodies give us. We live in a busy world: work, family, friends, and finances all take their important place and have their unique demands. Sometimes they become more important than our self-care. If we take the time to reconnect with our inner healing wisdom, we can tap into the resources of emotion, memory, and imagery. Then an awakened sense of wholeness is found, and we can activate this mind/body connection to support our immune system and promote healing.

What we think and feel directly impacts our health. Research has demonstrated that mind power can translate to muscle power. In a fascinating study, medical researchers in the Department of Psychology at University College in London, England, explained the health benefits of the physical activity involved with the work to the hospital cleaning staff. Once understood, the employees lost body fat, decreased their blood pressure, and increased their lean muscle mass. Their activity levels did not change. The only difference was what they were told about the health benefits of their work. Researchers concluded that increased mental awareness accounted for the health gains.

Sadly, many healthcare professionals summarily dismiss this as the placebo effect, the well-documented fact that sustained positive outcomes can be observed in response to treatment with a sugar pill or inert treatment versus actual medication. The nocebo effect is related. This refers to an undesirable effect being observed after receiving a placebo. Neither the placebo nor nocebo responses are biochemically generated. They are attributed solely to the recipient's optimistic or pessimistic beliefs and expectations.

Both the placebo and nocebo effects are very real. For cancer patients, if and when patients believe in a treatment, that belief itself nurtures health. Of course, the opposite is also true.

Your mind can be effectively employed in your quest for healing. By visualizing thoughts, images, and pictures of healing through use of the imagination, your body's defense mechanisms respond. Cortisol levels that inhibit maximum immune function drop. Endorphin levels rise, indicating increased immune activity.

In my own case, I came to believe my mind/body disciplines as more important than medicine. I employed the phrase, "I am cancer-free, a picture of health." Concurrently I would imagine myself vital and alive, arms outstretched overhead, reaching to the clear blue skies, and a big smile on my face.

I ask you to employ something similar. Or you may wish to seek the help of being guided by someone, either in person or by listening to a recording. The point is the mind/body connection can be triggered through visualization, guided imagery, and affirmation.

Although these techniques and modalities enhance the mind/body effect, simply listening to and honoring what your body is telling you to do is a good start. For example, fatigue is the single most common symptom of people with cancer. From the perspective of integrated cancer care, fatigue is your body's way of telling you to rest and to take time for self-care. Listen to what your body is telling you. Feel your energy level, and adjust your activity levels accordingly.

As you quiet your mind and deepen the intimate connection with your body, you will hear what your body is telling us. I am asking you to mobilize your mind, to listen to and nurture your body's healing wisdom. It is a powerful source of health.

You will find examples of three visualization exercises in the Resources section of this book.

Physical Exercise: The Five-Hour Standard

"I'm too tired."

"It's not fun."

"I don't have the time."

"My legs look ugly in gym shorts."

"The weather's bad."

You've heard them. I've used them. They are excuses for people who don't want to exercise. But even the very best of integrated cancer care will not be maximized without regular exercise. Think of it as a mandatory requirement.

In 2005, the *Journal of the American Medical Association* published a study on physical activity and survival after a cancer diagnosis. The study found that exercising just one hour per week could lower the risk of recurrence by approximately 20 percent. But the risk of recurrence was reduced by 50 percent when the exercise time was increased to three to five hours per week.

The benefits of exercise before, during, and after cancer treatment are now appearing frequently in medical research. When we started our work over a quarter-century ago, Cancer Recovery Group was the first organization to document the link between exercise and recovery. At that time, we did not clearly understand how much exercise and what type. Today, the answers are much clearer. And the answer is that you and I need to make daily exercise a part of our lives.

Cancer and its treatments cause significant changes in the body, including fatigue, muscle weakness, and loss of flexibility, which can result in normal daily activities becoming challenging. Movement counters these changes and becomes a key aspect of recovery and healing. Something as simple as gentle range of motion exercises following surgery will enhance energy, increase flexibility, improve mood, and often produce an overall feeling of greater well-being.

Mild exercise such as a brisk walk, house-cleaning, or gardening improves quality of life, sleep, and appetite. Moderate exercise also reduces the risks of heart disease, high blood pressure, diabetes, osteoporosis, anxiety, and depression.

At our affiliate Breast Cancer Charities of America, we have helped set the aerobic standard for minimum exercise at twenty to forty minutes three to five times per week. In 2006, a study found this level to be safe for cancer patients receiving chemotherapy. From our survivor interviews, we know that only 30 percent of cancer patients meet that standard. I am asking you to join that select group. And I am further encouraging you to work up to and maintain the high end of the standard, five hours per week.

You owe it to yourself to schedule a walk each and every day. Or perhaps you prefer gentle yoga or qigong, both of which combine relaxation and exercise. I ask you to exercise out-of-doors whenever possible. The fresh air and the exposure to sunlight are sources of health on their own.

The physiology of regular moderate exercise facilitates the flow of lymphatic fluid. This means our immune system can deal more effectively with the many toxins, bacteria, and abnormal cells. Unlike the circulatory system, which relies on the heart to pump the blood, the lymphatic system has no pump. Instead, lymph function relies on contraction of our muscles during our activities of daily living and exercise to move lymphatic fluid through the system. Moderate exercise also helps minimize lymphedema in cancer patients. This is the often painful fluid buildup many patients experience post-surgery and especially following removal of lymph nodes. Researchers examined the association between lymphedema and exercise and found that upper body weight training did not increase the risk of lymphedema—it helped. It is reasonable to conclude that cancer patients can and should engage in moderate upper body resistance training. In addition to exercise, and to support maximum lymph function, drinking at least eight glasses of water per day helps provide the needed hydration that optimizes lymphatic volume and fluid.

As much as I strive to make the message of this book gentle, personal, and filled with hope, I now need to deliver a short but loving lecture: take these exercise guidelines very seriously. The costs of failing to exercise are simply too great. Start slow. Find the right routine. Do something every day—no excuses.

Just do it! Join me in making daily exercise a central part of your life. Soon it will become more than a requirement, it will become a pleasure. And then you will know you are truly on the path to health and healing.

Nutrition: The Most Healthful Choice

A cancer diagnosis signals the time to launch an extreme nutritional makeover. It starts by eating actual food—that means quality, real natural food. If it is boxed or bottled or canned or packaged, be skeptical. A nutrition makeover means asking questions as you shop. How fresh are these ingredients? Where was it grown? Is it local? Is it organic? What does this label tell me? Does this contain genetically modified ingredients? What about sugar, particularly high-fructose corn syrup?

The cancer patient's guide to nutrition is simple and easily implemented. The best foods are predominantly fresh and organically grown fruits, vegetables, whole grains, and legumes. We also favor beans, nuts, and seeds. Select fish, some soy and soy alternatives, and egg whites in their natural form. It is preferable if the source of these foods is local.

What you are seeking is the wholesome foods that nature provides. This means to avoid processed foods, refined foods, and those that contain chemicals and additives. It also means we spend a great deal of our time shopping for food in the produce section of our market.

Cancer remains much less prevalent in cultures that continue to eat the unrefined foods of our ancestors. While modern technology has enabled us to mass-produce foods for high yields, long shelf life, and maximum profits, it is clear the nutritional values have been compromised in the process. Factory farming has changed the health integrity of our food. As a result, most people are missing essential nutrients that were commonplace in previous generations.

I am not asking you to go on a diet. I am asking you to change and improve your lifestyle. If you think you are going on a diet, chances are that you'll go off that diet. Sooner or later, for most people, being on a diet—any diet—is simply not sustainable. The word "diet" itself conjures up images of deprivation and restrictions. Nobody wants to be deprived and restricted, especially in the midst of a cancer diagnosis.

In contrast, I am asking you to adopt high nutrition as a wonderful way of life. The nutrition program explained in this book gives you maximum choices that taste *good*. It is satisfying and nutritious. And most important, it fights cancer.

In his book *Food Rules*, Michael Pollan brilliantly distills the nutrition discussion into seven words. He says, "Eat food. Not too much. Mostly plants." This should be the focal point of your nutrition program.

Eat food. Not the highly processed, nutritionally void, prepackaged foods so commonly found in most grocery stores. Instead, eat real, live, high-quality food. Pollan gives powerful advice when he says, "It's not food if it arrived through the window of your car."

Not too much. This is portion control. And unless you are in the wasting stages of cancer where you simply cannot maintain weight, the Scottish guideline "A little with quiet is the only diet" serves you well. Yet the good thing about a plant-based program is that you can eat more—up to ten servings a day of fresh vegetables and fruit.

Mostly plants. Not exclusively plants but predominantly plants—whole foods that are organically grown and filled with the thousands of natural phytonutrients that help create health and healing.

While there are few "thou shalt nots" in the Cancer Recovery nutrition program, there is one that I insist upon: cutting out sugar and the processed foods that contain these sugars. Avoid all artificial or chemical sweeteners such as sorbitol, xylitol, and mannitol. When you find it necessary to sweeten foods or drinks, use stevia, a natural herb, which can be used freely. This sweetener is now widely available in liquid, powder, or tablet form. Just ask at your local market. See the section of this book entitled "Cancer and Sugar" for a detailed analysis of this issue.

Finally, add generous amounts of health-enhancing superfoods. Superfoods are comprised of plants that have extraordinary anticancer effects. These include various kinds of cabbage, broccoli, garlic, several kinds of mushrooms, the right kind of soy, green tea, turmeric, raspberries, blueberries, strawberries, certain nuts, several herbs and spices, and even small amounts of dark chocolate.

Know this: healthful food is one of the primary sources of health and healing. What you eat is central to your recovery from cancer. Food's influence is considerable—every day, three times a day—for either speeding up or slowing down cancer growth. I urge you to take this nutritional guidance very seriously. Eating unhealthfully is simply too big a risk if you wish to recover from cancer.

Where do we find health? How can we know healing? It's right before us. And many cancer patients, in the rush to find a new conventional or complementary treatment, overlook the true sources that make for health and healing. The elements we have explored here are essential aspects of self-care. They help you create health and facilitate healing. Without these strong foundations, even the most exotic cancer treatments will crumble.

Health is more than healthcare. We simply must do more than treat the illness. We must create wellness.

CAUTION:
OVERTREATMENT

Too often it is a family member of a cancer patient who will turn to us at the Foundation when they observe that their loved one is becoming weakened and fragile. Often they fear the patient can withstand no more treatment. Weekly we hear heartbreaking stories like, "Radiation has my husband so fatigued he had to crawl to the bathroom." Or, "We just cannot go through the horror of another round of chemotherapy." The sad fact is we spend a great deal of time and effort helping cancer patients deal with overtreatment.

I became vividly aware of overtreatment in the early 1990s. A young California mother by the name of Nelene Fox turned to us for guidance. She had advanced invasive ductal carcinoma and asked if we could help her raise the $250,000 needed for a bone marrow transplant. Her insurance provider, Health Net, refused to cover the procedure because they considered it unproven and experimental.

Those were brutal days in cancer treatment. Oncologists boldly proclaimed that high-dose chemotherapy followed by bone marrow transplant offered the cure for advanced breast cancer. And medical journalists, especially the major weekly news magazines, blindly fanned the flames of this optimism. Many in the cancer community proclaimed high-dose chemo and bone marrow transplant to be the Holy Grail.

The procedure was exceedingly dangerous. I retain a newspaper clipping of one doctor describing the process: "We bring the patient to death's door through an intensive pre-transplant regimen of chemotherapy and radiation. Our treatment involves a four-drug regimen and is 35 to 40 percent more intensive than the regimens used in the recently reported studies. We administer our regimen in a highly specialized transplant unit, not in the outpatient setting. Although the treatment itself is associated with a 21-percent mortality rate, the payoff may be a higher proportion of women surviving and being cancer-free." Brutal by any standards.

While trying to persuade Health Net to pay, Nelene Fox raised the funds to have the procedure. But eight months later she died. Her brother, Mark Hiepler, an attorney, brought suit against his sister's insurance company. In what was considered a landmark case, he won. The jury awarded the Fox family $89 million. The case is considered a watershed moment in that thereafter most health insurance companies began approving high-dose chemotherapy with bone marrow transplant for advanced breast cancer.

This era spawned a desperate flurry of activities that attempted to position this procedure as the quintessential answer to cancer. With the financial help of the nation's biggest pharmaceutical companies, transplant doctors testified before Congress and appeared before the media. Advocacy groups like the Susan G. Komen Breast Cancer Foundation, now called Susan G. Komen for the Cure, lobbied both federal authorities and state legislatures to mandate insurance coverage for the procedure. Hospitals from coast to coast proudly rushed to equip their facilities with bone marrow transplant units, encouraging their physicians to learn the procedure. Transplanting cancer patients was good business.

At that time, Cancer Recovery Foundation was based in Southern California, where we ran the largest cancer support group in the nation. We always built our message around less-toxic and least-invasive prevention and treatment options. But in the early 1990s our message was drowned out. For nearly five years, the number one request from patients and their family members was information on high-dose chemo and bone marrow transplant.

New drugs were introduced that made it possible to harvest marrow cells from blood rather than having to extract it from a woman's hip. And soon it was possible to administer high-dose chemo and transplant on an outpatient basis. All systems were "go" to make high-dose chemotherapy and bone marrow transplant the new standard of care. Its efficacy was accepted as an article of faith.

We were located near the University of California–Irvine Medical Center. Their oncologists were only too happy to accommodate our organization's requests for presentations. And the transplanters were considered the ultimate authorities. Soon their lectures were filled to capacity. And the presentations went beyond metastatic breast cancer to suggest transplants had application in women with early-stage breast cancer—making for a larger market. It was not long thereafter that we received a report on the first application of the procedure in ovarian cancer, even though there was no evidence to support this use. High-dose chemotherapy followed by bone marrow transplant was the emerging model for all cancers.

I sat on the community advisory board of the hospital's cancer center. Prior to one meeting there was an animated discussion that transplants could be used for advanced prostate cancer. Finally the center's director, Dr. Frank Meyskens, Jr., quietly pointed out that advanced prostate cancer rarely responds to chemotherapy, no matter how high the dose.

It wasn't until 1999 at an American Society of Clinical Oncology (ASCO) meeting that researchers presented four studies that showed women did no better with the high-dose chemotherapy and bone marrow transplant treatment than those who received only low-dose chemotherapy. From that point forward, the procedure was discredited and today is largely abandoned.

MORE IS NOT BETTER

The beliefs behind the more-treatment mind-set die hard. And clinging to that worldview is why so much unnecessary care is delivered by doctors and hospitals. In the world of cancer, it is widely agreed that surgery is the most effective treatment, contributing more to halting the progression of the disease than the other treatment modalities combined. Yet beyond surgery, there is little certainty about which drugs or which procedures actually work best.

Our culture seeks cures. Most people in developed societies believe fervently in the doctrine that modern medicine cures. Cure—it's almost a statement of faith, pervasive on every continent. And most cancer patients look to its high priests, the oncologists, as their saviors. We seldom question the ongoing march of science. In fact, we expect it, taking scientific progress as a given. Both patients and healthcare professionals are deeply in need of believing that medicine cures and is safe.

This is exacerbated by the "Hammer Syndrome," something I first explored over twenty years ago. The syndrome looks like this: If you are a surgeon, every answer looks like surgery. If you are a radiation oncologist, all your answers point toward radiation. And if you are a medical oncologist, every answer involves drugs. Essentially, if you are trained in a narrow subspecialty, that's what you see as the answer. If you're a hammer, the whole world looks like a nail and you go around looking for nails to pound.

But there is much more to this overtreatment warning. Most oncologists lack the specialized training needed to independently interpret the evidence that is available to them. This leads even well-intentioned physicians to treat out of an understandable altruistic and humanitarian motive to help, even when they may not know what is the best thing to do based on actual outcomes.

Medical oncologists are famous for statements like, "We will never know if this drug can help you unless we do just one more round." There is a vast array of evidence to point out the last round is often the fatal round. And it is widely believed that thousands of patients die each year not from the cancer but from cancer treatment. It's called treatment-related mortality, or fatal adverse events (FAEs) and is typically discussed only in quiet whispers within the confines of doctors' lounges in America's hospitals.

In a series of 2010–2011 articles, the prestigious *Journal of the American Medical Association* again brought to the attention of the physician community the seriousness of FAEs. The editors included detailed focus on the new drug Avastin. Originally thought to be helpful in marginally prolonging life in patients with colorectal cancer, non-small cell lung cancer, and kidney cancer, the drug was now being touted and tested for the lucrative breast cancer market.

But in November of 2011, the FDA, the agency in the United States responsible for approval of pharmaceutical drugs, revoked the use of Avastin for breast cancer. The drug was linked to severe high blood pressure, internal bleeding, hemorrhaging, heart attack, heart failure, and death. Despite vocal protests by dozens of breast cancer groups and patients who claimed Avastin "saved their lives," the FDA withdrew approval because the drug, at best, prolonged life but also led to unacceptably high rates of FAEs.

It is interesting to note that in the United States many health insurance companies refused to pay for all or part of the costs of Avastin because of the low ratio of benefits to cost. In countries with national health systems, such as the UK and Canada, the healthcare systems restricted its use for the same reasons. The drug's manufacturer, Genentech, which charged up to $100,000 per year per patient, stood by its claims that the cost of Avastin was justified and the drug was effective.

In the mid-1990s, my wife and I personally walked through a cancer experience with Denise, a close family friend. After the oncologist delivered Denise's diagnosis and reviewed the recommended treatment protocol, the kindly, soft-spoken, and well-meaning oncologist pulled me aside and said, "Your friend is in for a rough time. We can give her a year, maybe a little more."

Denise and her family had blind faith in medicine and wanted to know all the "newest" treatment options. The answer was some early-stage clinical trials. I tried to explain the dangers of early-stage clinical trials, as well as the limits of chemotherapy, to our friends. But Denise's answer was always, "Let's try." At the end of her battle, the kindly doctor said, "We need to try this new drug. It's a shot in the dark. But we'll never know unless we try."

She never made it out of the hospital alive. Her mother shared Denise's medical records with me, including the autopsy report. There we found the words "death not due to disease progression," which is medical code for overtreatment. Denise was another victim.

In America, the fear of malpractice drives what is euphemistically called "defensive medicine." This is the practice of diagnostic and therapeutic procedures conducted primarily as a safeguard against possible malpractice liability, not as a means to improve a patient's health. In cancer, fear of litigation is often behind a long list of diagnostic scans, genetic tests, specialty surgeries, and treatment recommendations involving radiation and chemotherapy, even when the cancer has been diagnosed at the very earliest stages.

Overtreatment may also be a result of the prevailing local medical practices. This phenomenon rests with the fact that the same types and stages of cancer are treated in very different ways in different geographic regions. Even when excellent outcomes evidence exists, treatment choices can and do vary dramatically from place to place.

This is clearly the case in early-stage breast cancer. Studies show that mastectomy and lumpectomy achieve similar long-term survival. But doctors differ sharply in their attitudes toward these treatments. John E. Wennberg, M.D., Ph.D., pointed out in the Dartmouth Atlas of Health Care studies that there are regions in the United States in which virtually no women covered by Medicare underwent lumpectomy, while in another, nearly half did.

Why such massive disparity? Clearly, it was not the science, as the studies show similar outcomes. Based on the science you could expect something closer to 50 percent mastectomies and 50 percent lumpectomies. But many treatment decisions are based on nothing more than the attitude of, "That's the way we treat here." As an informed cancer patient, it is critical that you understand whether local customs, rather than the best medicine, may be driving your treatment recommendations. Check the Dartmouth Atlas, www.dartmouthatlas.org, to be sure.

Such extreme variations arise because patients commonly and willingly delegate decision-making to their physicians. Decision delegation is most often given under the assumption that the doctor knows best. Behind it is a belief that physicians can always understand a patient's values and thus recommend what is the most appropriate treatment for each person. But often, very often, local custom rather than outcomes-based evidence drives these treatment recommendations. Studies show that when patients are fully informed about their options, they often choose very differently from their physicians.

Beyond all these very understandable reasons, I have come to believe that the most powerful reason American doctors and hospitals overtest and overtreat is that most of them are paid for how *much* care they deliver rather than how *well* they take care of their patients. Western medicine, especially as practiced in the United States, is largely reimbursed on a piece-rate basis. It's like the man on the old-fashioned assembly line; the more widgets he made, the more he was paid. This one factor alone has led to a massive overtreatment of many illnesses, including cancer, and especially breast and prostate cancers.

I understand this next statement is harsh—but absolutely true. To better understand much of cancer treatment, *follow the money*.

Hospitals, doctors, medical equipment manufacturers, pharmaceutical companies, and all the organizations that derive their revenue from cancer diagnosis and treatment have a bias. They have a deeply vested interest in the more-treatment-is-better-treatment paradigm. Pharmaceutical companies do not want medical oncologists to prescribe less chemotherapy. Manufacturers of radiology equipment do not promote the use of less radiation. And the companies that manufacture surgical gloves do not want fewer surgeries. It goes on and on and on.

OVERTREATING BREAST CANCER AND PROSTATE CANCER

If you have been diagnosed with either breast or prostate cancer, be especially careful of overtreatment. These are the two most overdiagnosed and overtreated cancers.

There is a raging debate around the question whether early-stage breast abnormalities, called ductal carcinoma in situ (DCIS), are actually cancer. These micro-calcifications come and go. With the newest digital mammography, DCIS can be tracked from their very earliest appearance. Most disappear on their own. Some do not. Most are benign. A very small percentage are malignant. The problem lies in the fact that current technology has no way of tracking whether they are cancerous unless a needle or tissue biopsy is performed. Current thinking and practice is to treat all DCIS as a possible malignancy. With that mind-set comes overtreatment and all the attendant complications.

The same experience is at work with prostate cancer. A blood test called the prostate specific antigen (PSA) measures a protein that is secreted by the prostate gland. High levels of this protein are often associated with the presence of prostate cancer and other prostate problems. But the PSA test is so imprecise that the U.S. Preventive Services Task Force declared, "Prostate-specific antigen-based screening results in small or no reduction in prostate cancer–specific mortality and is associated with harms related to subsequent evaluation and treatments, some of which may be unnecessary."

Yet current thinking and practice is to consider a PSA level of 4 ng/mL as a possible malignancy. In actuality, current medical technology has no way of determining if the prostate is malignant unless a needle or tissue biopsy is performed, once again leading to unnecessary treatments.

My suggestion with suspicions of both early-stage breast cancer and early-stage prostate cancer is "active surveillance." For suspected breast cancer, this means three clinical breast exams followed by a mammogram over six months and a subsequent comparison of the results. For suspected prostate cancer, this means three PSA tests over six months and a subsequent comparison of those results. Provided there are no other symptoms, the six-month time frame is not too long to wait if treatment is needed. Six months is also an adequate time frame to compare tests and determine if there is a natural regression in the initially suspicious results.

As you set foot on the cancer journey, be very aware. Overdiagnosis and overtreatment are hidden parts of the system. You are not looking for more medicine, you are seeking the best medicine. The two are not the same. This book will guide you in that quest.

Chemotherapy: Be Skeptical

In nearly three decades of experience in this field, nowhere in the world of cancer is there more overtreatment than with chemotherapy. At Cancer Recovery Foundation, we receive more calls and e-mails involving the subject of chemotherapy than all other inquiries combined.

First, I wish to make it clear to all who read this that I am not a fan of chemotherapy. I am very cautious, even skeptical, about this treatment modality. I want you to know of my belief—some have called it a blind bias—and then ask you to balance it with your own research and convictions regarding your cancer treatment choices.

Make no mistake: chemotherapy is exceedingly dangerous, even when administered by the most experienced oncologists. It is a chemical, a cytotoxin, a poison. Simply put, the goal of chemotherapy is to harm cancer cells by poisoning them in order to disrupt their ability to grow and multiply. Sometimes, in some cases of cancer, it works.

However, in this process your host defense system is poisoned, typically compromised, and, at high doses, often irreparably damaged. Further, tumors that initially respond to treatment frequently develop a resistance to these toxic drugs. And while a tumor may respond a second time, the response is often at a much lower level of effectiveness.

Worse, with longer-term treatment, the body is typically weakened to a point where less-invasive alternatives have little chance to effectively rebuild immune function, extend life, or yield quality-of-life gains.

I initially raised my concerns about chemotherapy in the first edition of this book. Since that time I have been relentless on the overuse of this treatment modality. Sadly, little has changed in the twenty years since that first warning. This treatment modality remains overused. It also underperforms. And all the while tens of thousands of patients are left with life-altering permanent disabilities.

Let me be clear. I want to state where chemotherapy has a place. Science shows chemotherapy to be efficacious in producing long-term remission in most cases of Hodgkin's disease, acute lymphocytic leukemia, and testicular cancer. Chemotherapy is also shown to be effective in a handful of relatively rare, mainly childhood cancers including Burkitt's lymphoma, lymphosarcoma, and choriocarcinoma. Used with surgery and/or radiation therapy, chemotherapy also plays a role in the successful treatment of Wilms' tumor, Ewing's sarcoma, rhabdomyosarcoma, and retinoblastoma.

In addition, research shows chemotherapy to be effective in extending life by several months in many cases of ovarian cancer and small-cell lung cancer. However, chemotherapy does not produce a cure.

Sadly, "adjuvant" (additional) chemotherapy has become the standard of care for many cancers. This is sad because the evidence is simply not conclusive. Breast cancer is a perfect example. At best, there may be a very small statistical advantage, at most a 2 to 4 percent point gain, in survival rates for those women who receive chemotherapy. This small gain must be weighed against the very real potential for collateral damage caused by the same treatment.

Among a class of chemotherapy drugs called anthrocyclines is one with the generic name Doxorubicin, better known under its most common brand name, Adriamycin, a product of Pfizer. In the back rooms of chemotherapy infusion bays this drug is called "Red Devil" and even "Red Death." The single most common long-term problem, in 10 to 15 percent of patients so treated, is compromised heart function, even congestive heart failure. In addition, the side effects typically include hair loss, mouth ulcers, dark urine, night sweats, insomnia, distortion in fingernails and toenails, muscle weakness, and extreme fatigue. The list goes on to even more serious side effects like lowered white blood cell counts, lowered red blood cell counts, and lower platelet counts—all at the critical time when these natural immune system components need to be at maximum functioning levels. In other words, while "Red Devil" may marginally increase survival rates, it substantially increases the risk of other serious life-threatening health problems.

For postmenopausal women with breast cancer, a statistically stronger case can be made for the hormone blocker raloxifene, now the preferred choice over tamoxifen. However, both these drugs have been linked to other health problems including blood clots, stroke, and increases in endometrial cancer, uterine cancer, and liver cancer.

As previously noted, chemotherapy's one other area of limited success is colon cancer. There is still no conclusive evidence of its effectiveness except after lymph-node involvement. Even then, the gain in life expectancy is months, not years, and quality of life typically suffers. Sadly, once again, even though the clinical evidence is at best mixed, the current Western practice says to treat with chemotherapy in virtually all cases of colon cancer.

After studying this carefully for over two decades, I believe oncologists who are trained in Western practices are administering chemotherapy to more patients, across a wider spectrum of malignant diseases, based on the hope it may show results. The cancer community has tended to extrapolate narrow successes and consider nearly all patients, especially those with metastatic or recurrent cancer, as candidates for chemotherapy. All this to the exclusion of high-level nutrition, moderate exercise, and mind/body regimens.

Once again, and despite my urgent warning, chemotherapy may have a role in your cancer treatment program, particularly if your diagnosis is one of the cancers that typically respond to the treatment. But please do not blindly accept the recommendation to undergo chemotherapy. Conduct your own investigation. Understand exactly what can and what cannot be expected from any recommendation. Only then should you decide.

STOPPING CHEMOTHERAPY: A CALL FOR A NEW STANDARD

Is there a time to stop chemotherapy? I believe there is. And I believe that time to be when there has been no demonstrated progress after three cycles of treatment.

We recently assisted a woman whose mother was having extensive quality of life difficulties with her chemotherapy treatments. In their last conversation with the doctor, he suggested they consider stopping chemotherapy because it was no longer effective and was causing so many side effects. However, her mother said she wanted to continue because she wanted to "keep on fighting." The woman asked, "How do we decide when to stop chemotherapy? And how do I talk to my mother?"

Obviously, this was a very sensitive conversation to have. But when an oncologist acknowledges that cancer treatment is no longer achieving results, it is not only time, but past time, to discontinue that treatment. And an excellent rule of thumb is that if there is no progress following three cycles, it is time to stop.

If you, or a loved one, are faced with this conundrum where treatment is not making a difference, ask key questions such as, "Is continuing treatment going to make a significant difference in stopping the progression of the cancer?" And, "If we discontinue treatment, can we expect the nausea, pain, and other discomforts to diminish?" If the doctor answers that treatment at this point will not make a significant difference in life expectancy but discontinuing it will improve quality of life, it is clearly time to stop.

Unfortunately, there is an exceedingly disturbing dark side to this issue. Thousands of oncologists urge as "best practice" the continuation of chemotherapy even when there is no response. As we previously discussed with treatment-related deaths and fatal adverse events, many treatments continue right until the patient dies. In the medical profession this is called "flogging," as in beating a dead horse.

The root of this problem is the fee-for-service reimbursement system under which most of Western medicine operates. And in no place is it more disturbing than end-of-life care. I realize that the culture in America also drives the "more treatment" mindset. Millions of people believe so deeply in medicine that sometimes we like to believe death itself is optional. And so treatment is continued. But when a patient is so sick they can't even raise their head off the pillow, another cycle of chemotherapy is absolutely not called for. I have witnessed just that too many times to count.

I now issue a clarion call to the oncology community to stop condoning this unethical practice. If after three cycles of treatment there is no progress, it is then time to stop. Thereafter, fully embrace the integrated cancer care options, especially nutrition, exercise, and the mind/body disciplines.

Chemotherapy has a cumulative effect. It often takes longer and longer to recover from failed treatments. But provided the patient's physical status has not deteriorated to incapacitation, integrated cancer care strategies may be able to help signifi-cantly. In fact, stopping chemotherapy treatment should be viewed not so much as "giving up" as it is "freeing one up" to embrace life and all the more natural alternatives that can lead to better days and more days. Just because one conventional treat-ment can no longer be expected to bring about a cure doesn't mean there are no other options. And this is certainly not time to give up hope.

Science says, "Show me the data." The data says, beyond the previously mentioned cancers where chemotherapy is efficacious, there is no proof of chemotherapy's effectiveness in the form of large-scale randomized clinical trials. The unvarnished truth is that the widespread use of chemotherapy is not based on con-vincing scientific data. Even in those cancers where positive out-comes can be observed, current chemotherapy regimens alone fail to produce a cure, a longer life, or improved quality of life. It is the multifaceted integrated cancer care approach empha-sized throughout this book that is crucial to understand and implement.

FRACTIONATED DOSE TREATMENT

Having stated my very real and urgent reservations, I need to add that chemotherapy may be right for you at some point in time. One important aspect of any treatment's success is the be-lief both the doctor and the patient bring to the process. It's un-derstandable that many oncologists believe in chemotherapy based on tumor response, or "shrinkage." Theoretically, it makes sense. If you can reduce the tumor burden, perhaps the body can rebuild immune function.

From the patient's viewpoint, it is also understandable. Since chemotherapy is widely accepted and supported by the medical community, since insurance will reimburse for its administration, and since billions of cancer research dollars are invested in inves-tigating this treatment modality, it comes with a great deal of up-front cultural support. With all that evidence, it seems believable despite its mediocre outcomes. And based on that belief alone it may have a place.

If you do choose this therapy, I urge you to use extreme caution in approving high-dose chemotherapy. There are now dozens of studies on the use of high-dose chemotherapy across a broad spectrum of cancers. The results are universally disappointing. There simply are very few studies that show better outcomes with high-dose chemotherapy compared to those receiving lower dose. This data directly challenges earlier studies and widely held assumptions among the cancer community's research elite regarding increased survival rates with higher doses.

Is there a middle ground you could choose? Fractionated dose chemotherapy, smaller doses infused over an extended period of time, is a good alternative. The toxic effects of the drugs are typically minimized because the lower doses do not create massive systemic toxicity. In fact, there exists an increasing body of evidence from Europe that low-dose chemotherapy appears to halt the growth of microscopic blood vessels that supply solid tumors. Other studies purport to show fractionated dose chemotherapy may result in actually stimulating immune function. Although most conventionally trained Western oncologists dismiss this evidence, I predict variations of this homeopathic "less-is-more" approach will become more widely accepted.

Finally, if you choose to undergo chemotherapy or have already had chemotherapy, study carefully this book's chapters on "Adopt This Nutritional Strategy During Treatment," #21, and "Determine Your Nutritional Supplement Program," #25. Start strengthening and rebuilding your immune system immediately.

When you analyze chemotherapy as a treatment for cancer, I beg you to understand the side effects, both short-term and long-term, and compare them to actual proven results. Then make your choice. If chemotherapy is started and if you are debilitated, confined to bed, or unable to eat, you not only have every right but you also have the responsibility to call a halt to treatment. Even in the face of threats and warnings from medical providers and family, continuing treatment or not is your personal decision.

In the final analysis, the vast majority of chemotherapy-based cancer treatments do not of themselves cure. My general guidance: surgery, yes. Radiation, maybe. Chemotherapy, no—or at least be skeptical, very skeptical indeed.

A
Road
Map to
Recovery

Learning from the True Experts

After my surgeon told me I had lung cancer and just thirty days to live, I was stunned. One moment I was in tears, the next I was enraged. I thought it was all a mistake, convinced my tests had been confused with another patient's. I was filled with fear and self-pity. One afternoon I yelled out loud, "Oh God, what can I do?"

That question was answered. No, God did not part the clouds and speak; I remain a committed skeptic regarding such claims. But figuratively, the clouds were parted and God did speak. It was nonverbal communication, a distinct impression that my task was to search for survivors. I became aware, vitally aware—a knowing—that I was to seek people who were "supposed" to die but had lived. And once I found them, I was to learn from their experience.

Over the years, I have interviewed and received surveys from over 16,000 survivors of "terminal" illness. These are the people who have been told the equivalent of "Get your affairs in order. You are about to die." They are the brave patients who, at one time, had no hope—the people the medical community wrote off. But these same people lived.

These inspiring individuals, who possess no more courage or ability than you or me, teach some very powerful lessons from which we would be well-served to learn. These ideas and practices have worked successfully for me and hundreds of thousands of other cancer patients. I am convinced these lessons and strategies can be pivotal in your life and your health.

After I conducted over 500 interviews, it became clear there were shared patterns to most of the individual outcomes. For example, the vast majority of survivors do not believe they recovered their health by chance or by being passive. The triumphant patients worked for their wellness, earning it on a daily basis. Neither do most cancer survivors credit their doctors alone, or even primarily, for their recovery. Instead, these exceptional patients focus on personally mobilizing body, mind, and spirit in their quest for high-level wellness.

Consistent patterns emerged from the survivor interviews. In 1988, I first summarized them and combined them into an eight-strategy program. In 2006, after thousands of additional interviews, I further refined them into six easily understood concepts that anyone could understand and put to use. Today, through Cancer Recovery Foundation International, over ten million people have used these principles as a road map, a strategic plan to enhance their health and enrich their lives. I want the same for you.

The Six Strategies

Before we come to the "50 Essential Things," I'd like to give you an overview of the six basic approaches that cancer survivors have in common. Here is what emerged from the survivor interviews.

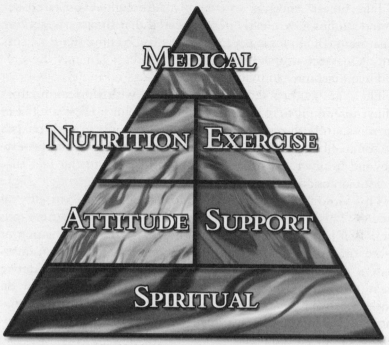

Strategy #1: Medical Treatment

Over 96 percent of cancer survivors start and complete at least one treatment program that is grounded in conventional medical care. Surgery, radiation therapy, chemotherapy, hormonal therapy, and immunotherapy—often in combination—are the treatments of choice. I was both surprised and encouraged by this.

Let me be very clear. Orthodox treatments have an important role in cancer survival. The overwhelming majority of cancer survivors do embrace conventional medical care. This is a very important message.

But there is a significant issue that has become much clearer since we first started our work. It's the gross inconsistency in the medical treatment prescribed for similar diagnoses.

Take breast cancer as an example. Although several well-designed studies have clearly demonstrated that Breast Conserving Treatment (BCT) for stage I and II disease has the same success rate as mastectomy, the removal of the breast remains the predominant treatment.

There are marked regional differences, with women in larger cities more likely to receive BCT than those in rural areas. There is even a study showing double mastectomy, where both breasts are removed even when cancer exists in only one, is the fastest-growing breast cancer treatment. All this despite the fact that the outcomes are statistically the same.

This same treatment inconsistency is seen across virtually all cancers. This is why patients everywhere must take matters into their own hands, demanding full knowledge and explanation of all treatment options. Thankfully, the amount of treatment information now available is significant. Demanding hard evidence regarding the effectiveness of suggested treatments is the key. So while 96 out of 100 surviving patients still opt for conventional treatments, their treatment decisions are more informed today than ever before. Do likewise.

Importantly, cancer survivors do not stop with conventional medical treatment. As you study the "50 Essential Things," you will see how survivors take charge of the management of their entire health and well-being. They choose doctors in whom they have confidence, often researching their educational background and clinical track record. Survivors consent only to treatment programs in which they have high confidence. Plus, survivors aggressively integrate complementary and alternative approaches with traditional medical care.

Survivors are active patients, involved with each decision, making certain they are fully informed and understand each component of their recovery program. Conventional medicine, yes. Patient control, even more. It is the prominent theme among cancer survivors.

Strategy #2: Nutrition

Following medical care, dietary changes are the most common strategy adopted by the cancer survivors. The increasing importance of nutrition in cancer recovery has been one of the most significant shifts in the last decade. No longer is the old "Eat whatever you want" theory widely accepted.

Today, viewing "food as medicine" is the norm among cancer survivors. The most common nutritional shifts are toward diets that feature the following:

- Whole foods
- Foods low in fat, salt, and sugar
- An emphasis on fresh vegetables, fresh fruits, and whole grains
- Pure water

The single major dietary shift is consuming foods that are less processed. If it is boxed or bottled or canned or packaged, the food comes under immediate suspicion. These prepared foods tend to deliver calories with less nutrition than their fresh counterparts. In practice, cancer survivors spend most of their grocery shopping time in the produce section of their local market.

Nutritional supplements, while not taking the place of a whole food diet, are widely employed by cancer survivors. While there exists a lack of consensus in actual practice, survivors widely recognize the role of vitamin, mineral, and herbal supplements in the management of cancer. Thankfully, better science is producing evidence to support nutrition as a central element in cancer recovery.

One other observation on nutrition: cancer survivors eat with awareness. There is a marked increase in "nutritional IQ" among cancer patients, especially over the past twenty years. Nutrition, not simply calories, has become the emerging battle cry of cancer patients in Western cultures. And survivors carry the attitude that a healthy diet is something they "get" to do, as opposed to something they "have" to do, to contribute to their survival. More specifics on nutrition will be found later in this book.

Strategy #3: Exercise

Survivors engage in some form of physical exercise virtually every day. Cancer Recovery Foundation was the first organization to document this trend over twenty years ago. It has accelerated. Today, the science is catching up with the survivors' practices and confirming the significant benefits of exercise.

Nearly nine out of ten cancer survivors I have interviewed and surveyed affirm the role of regular physical exercise in their own journey. I talked to bikers, swimmers, joggers, and walkers—lots of walkers. A brisk twenty-minute walk each day, with moderate strength training every other day, seems to be ideal. Do you know what? That's something all of us can do.

Most inspiring are the patients who started exercise programs even while confined to hospitals beds or wheelchairs. In spite of physical limits, these people exercised. If you seek to overcome cancer, physical exercise needs to be an important part of your program.

Strategy #4: Attitude

Survivors believe they will survive. Survivors embrace beliefs that generate attitudes and, in turn, create emotions that nurture healing. This is the mind-body connection. It is powerful.

Do beliefs and attitudes actually heal? Survivors see a direct link. They choose beliefs and attitudes about illness and wellness that empower. The most fundamental and empowering belief is that cancer does not mean death. It's sad but true that much of the world still considers cancer and death to be synonymous. Survivors emphatically reject that belief.

This does not translate into denial, or some "be-positive-against-all-evidence" thinking. It's a warrior's attitude that survivors demonstrate. There is a marked tough-mindedness in the cancer survivor community—"feistiness," as actress Suzanne Somers once described it. You see it everywhere.

Survivors face this truth: cancer may or may not mean death. This set of beliefs and attitudes results in emotions that carry vastly different outlooks from either the super-positive or hopelessly negative cancer patients. "Yes, I may die," said Chris Winters, a thirty-something California housewife. "But I am going to live to the fullest with cancer. I am not going to die of fear and hopelessness."

I want you to know that Chris's attitude is the essence of survivorship. These essential beliefs extend to medical treatments and potential side effects. Survivors envision their treatments as highly effective. They further believe side effects will be minimal and manageable. The "50 Essential Things" will help you understand and apply these attitudes of healing to your own integrated cancer care program.

You will not be surprised to learn that survivors believe they have the absolute central role in the recovery process. This belief and resulting attitude is at complete odds with millions of other cancer patients who defer virtually every question to their doctors. Not survivors.

It's surprising: survivors have interesting relationships with their medical team. They want the best of care and respect those healthcare professionals who speak truth, patiently explaining what evidence supports their treatment recommendations and what outcomes can be expected. But if that information is not freely forthcoming, survivors can be exceptionally confrontational. Survivors check and recheck physician recommendations, often challenging tests, treatments, and prognoses. Many survivors change doctors in search of those who can be trusted and who meet their expectations.

Strategy #5: Support

Relationships. Survivors invest time and emotional energy in relationships that nurture. They also invest less time and energy in relationships that are toxic. While this may seem to be a benign practice, it has some surprising holistic health implications.

Loving relationships with friends, relatives, lovers, spouses, children, coworkers, and employees—or the lack of those relationships—build us up or tear us down. Survivors become "relationship sensitive," examining, perhaps for the first time in their lives, how they relate to other people. It is quite common for survivors to put difficult relationships on hold, especially during any debilitating treatment phase. This does not mean survivors exile toxic people from their lives for all time. But it certainly signals reduced emotional and even spiritual investment in those relationships.

Cancer gives patients permission to examine a wide variety of life choices, especially their network of social support. Changes are often made. That is helpful because much of the work of getting well again takes place within the patient's social support network. The last thing a cancer patient needs is a critical person second-guessing every decision or predicting ultimate doom.

New and important research is now demonstrating the health benefits of supportive relationships. As much as I wish the research extended to the health benefits of cancer support groups, it currently does not show conclusive proof of benefits. But this much we know to be true of support: survivors have at least one person with whom they can share everything, literally everything, without fear of judgment. That is a powerful healing elixir.

Strategy #6: Spiritual

Cancer survivors embrace a more spiritual perspective. They repeatedly speak of seeing life differently now compared to before their brush with death. This spiritual outlook stands in marked contrast to other cancer patients who obsess over a body that may be riddled with disease or endlessly mourn over dreams that are hopelessly derailed. Survivors surprise me in that they always seem to be able to grasp the high value of "now"—the simple and readily available life that is theirs even in spite of cancer. "I have today," said Doris, a fifty-year-old colon cancer patient. "That's a lot to be grateful for."

To label spirituality a "strategy" is inadequate. Survivors tend to undergo a spiritual transformation that is quite deep. For thousands of people, it becomes the central focus of their entire lives. In essence, they become new people.

This more spiritual perspective is not an issue of religion. Many survivors reject traditional religious practices. It's an old adage: just because you sit in a garage does not mean you will become a car. And just because you sit in a church does not mean you will become more spiritual. Clearly, no single doctrine or creed brings prepackaged answers.

Nor does this spirituality simply consist of bland platitudes. Instead, the transformation is typically seen as actively cultivating an inner peace, a serenity, a quiet confidence, a more grateful and joyful way of living. In a very real sense, survivors have come to let God work in and through them. Marianne Kegan, an ovarian cancer survivor, explained the essential nature of the spiritual walk. She said, "Now, when I walk into a room, I am there serving as God's representative." For millions of cancer survivors, this is the apex of the healing journey.

IMPLEMENTATION INTELLIGENCE

Each of these six strategies is important and essential to cancer survival. However, they are not always equal. Timing is an issue. If the decision is made to consider and commence medical treatment, nearly all the emphasis tends to be placed on that area. Once in place, survivors let the doctors treat while they focus on nutrition, exercise, attitude, and the holistic aspects of getting well again.

Implementation of one principle typically follows another at the appropriate time. Few survivors make simultaneous wholesale changes. Those who do attempt to change too much too quickly often meet with temporary defeat and have to start again.

Many survivors note that solving a relationship issue may have been just as important in their recovery as medical treatment. Adopting a healthy nutritional program and making a commitment to daily exercise may be on par with the contribution of radiation or chemotherapy.

It takes us back to where we started. We first review our state of health. That state is a result of the many interactive components of body, mind, and spirit. Yes, cell biology may be a component, but it is more often the result, the end game, of a host of other lifestyle choices.

Nearly all survivors agree it is the balance, the comprehensive integrated approach, that makes for survivorship. The survivors believe they have earned their return to health, aligning themselves with their own immense healing capacity. "Healing springs from within," said Randall Washington. "I simply had to work with God to release it."

Let's summarize to this point. The integration of these six key strategies represented by the cancer survival pyramid creates the framework for the cancer recovery process:

Medical	Attitude
Nutrition	Support
Exercise	Spiritual

The cancer survival pyramid is the context, the strategic plan, in which the "50 Essential Things" are implemented. The pyramid is your big picture, your road map. Consult it often.

Part Two

The
50
Essential
Things
to Do

The First Step: Understand Your Diagnosis

Your number one priority following a cancer diagnosis is to put in place the best integrated cancer care program you can possibly design. This is much more than simply going to one doctor and saying, "Treat me."

The decisions you make regarding your cancer care and recovery program are some of the most important you will make in your entire life. Begin the journey through cancer by following this course of action, which has proven highly effective for hundreds of thousands of cancer survivors.

#1

STOP
"AWFULIZING"

You've been told "It's cancer." I have deep compassion for you. I fully appreciate your feelings. I've been there, too.

First, you're in shock and filled with fear. The next moment you're angry but not quite certain at what or whom. Then comes the thoughts of, "How did this happen? Why me?" Even the guilt starts to creep in, "Did I bring this on myself?" Plus all the questions have started to rush through your mind: "Will I die?" "How long do I have?" "What will happen to my family?" And on and on and on. Your mind is overwhelmed at times.

Be calm. Try not to panic. I know that this is easier said than done. But be aware that panic will only inhibit rational and positive action.

Cancer is a serious illness, but it is not necessarily fatal. You do have the luxury of some time. Unlike a severed artery, cancer does not require you to do something this very instant. A hurried response, based in the emotions of fear and panic, is neither required nor preferred. In fact, a hurried response may be harmful. Don't take that as a license for inaction, however.

Stop and examine your frenzied thoughts for just a moment. It is at the beginning stages of this journey that clear decision-making will be most important. With these early decisions, you will ensure that your illness is properly treated. Panic acts only to your detriment.

Panic is a mental phenomenon, a response to our beliefs about cancer being frightful and overpowering. The process can accurately be labeled as "awfulizing." Isn't that an apt description? When we awfulize, we mentally take our current situation to its worst possible conclusion.

If we will objectively observe our emotions for just a moment, we will see something different from initial appearances. The intense panic that virtually every cancer patient experiences is actually the mind projecting its fears about the unknown future. Think about it, and understand this truth: Panic is caused by the mind. It's an assumption. It is not based on material fact.

Our fear-filled thoughts do not necessarily determine our future. We have a choice. This is a profound healing insight.

What to do when you start to feel anxious emotions arising inside? Try to witness them. Just observe. You may want to give those emotions an image. View them, and yourself, in your mind's eye. Instead of putting yourself in the role of a victim who is hopelessly caught in a web of panic and despair, become the observer. By not engaging the mind in battle, by simply watching the emotions and letting go, your panic will soon subside.

For example, Gwen Clement said she gave her fears a name. She would catch herself becoming anxious and say, "Hey, Mr. Fear. What are you doing here? Get out of my life." Then she would replace that fear with a short prayer of gratitude. "Thank you, God, for giving me long life."

I encourage you to do the same, to develop your version of speaking to your fears, to literally tell them to go away. Then always end by imagining yourself as a victor. Give yourself an image of a competent and confident person who is about to make some very important choices. Clear decision-making can and will be yours.

An Essential Thing to Do

Sit down. Take a deep breath. Say out loud, "Cancer does not mean death." Observe your emotions. Detach by separating who you are as a person from the emotional panic you may be feeling. You are not uncontrolled fear even though you may be experiencing fear. Understand that difference. Then immediately read and act on the next two essential things to do.

#2

TAKE CHARGE

Who is the most important person on your cancer recovery team? Some people believe it is their surgeon. Others believe it is their oncologist. Some choose the medical or diagnostic technicians, others the nurses, and still others choose their spouse.

But the most important person on your cancer recovery team is you! You are the one who is ill. It is you who must work to get well again. You are the character of central importance. And you need to put yourself in charge.

Millions of cancer patients surrender leadership of their recovery program way too often and way too willingly. Elizabeth Smalley, a thirty-eight-year-old housewife, was diagnosed with breast cancer. Her treatment was not progressing as expected, and the side effects depleted her. It all left Elizabeth understandably discouraged. Her doctor kept assuring her, "We're doing all we can. Trust me."

Following an especially difficult week, Elizabeth asked herself, "Do I accept the course of this treatment or do I try something new?" She called and made an appointment at a comprehensive cancer center that was a four-hour drive from her home. Doctors there recommended a different treatment program. Elizabeth took back that recommendation to her home doctor for implementation. "Personally taking charge was my turning point," explained a healthy Elizabeth four years after her bold and assertive decision.

Survivors take charge. View yourself as the manager of a baseball team or whatever organizational analogy you like. This is your cancer recovery team. The team's mission is to get you well again. You'll want a strong starting pitcher; many times that is a nutritionist or an oncologist. And you'll need many other team members: a catcher, infielders, outfielders. Equate these with specialists. You, the manager, choose the team that is on the field at any given moment.

Traditionally, consumers play a passive role in the healthcare system, going along with virtually whatever doctors and allied healthcare professionals recommend. We're encouraged to consent. Is that why we're called "patients"? This passive attitude does not serve you well. Decide you will take charge now!

An Essential Thing to Do

Evaluate your team. Who are the players? Who is managing this team? Is it a one-person show? How many more people could be helping? Are the team members working for you? Do some seem to be working against you? One woman remarked, "Every time I go to the doctor, I feel like I am in enemy territory." If you feel that way, you need to make a substitution. Remember: You are in charge!

#3

Ask Your Doctor These Questions

It is critically important for you to clearly understand your cancer diagnosis and proposed treatment plan. An important part of managing your care is knowing what questions to ask your doctor. Here are some examples of the types of questions you will want to ask your doctor:

Overview

- Precisely what type of cancer do I have?
- Where exactly is it located?
- What are my risks if I do not treat this disease?
- Is this type of cancer caused by genetic factors? Are other members of my family at risk?

Symptoms

- What are the most common symptoms of this type of cancer?
- Is there anything that can be done to make my symptoms or side effects better?

- Are there activities that may make them worse?
- If new symptoms or side effects arise or existing ones worsen, what should I do?

Diagnosis

- What diagnostic tests have you performed? What further tests are necessary?
- What information will these tests tell us?
- How can I prepare myself for each test or procedure?
- Where do I need to go to have these tests?
- When will I get the results? How will the results be communicated to me?
- Will you explain, in patient-friendly language, the pathology report to me?
- Is there any indication a second pathology report is necessary?
- If I seek a second opinion, will I have to repeat any tests or procedures?

Staging

- What is the stage of my cancer? In patient-friendly language, what does this mean?
- Has cancer spread to my lymph nodes or anywhere else?
- How is staging used to determine my cancer treatment?

Treatment

- What are my treatment options?
- Which treatments, or combination of treatments, do you recommend? Why?
- What is the goal of the treatment plan you are recommending?
- Who will be part of my treatment team? What does each member do?
- How much experience do you and the treatment team have treating this type of cancer?
- Will I need to be hospitalized for treatment or is this treatment done in an outpatient setting?

- What is the expected timeline for my treatment plan?
- How will this treatment affect my daily life? Will I be able to work, exercise, and perform my usual activities?
- What are the short-term side effects of this cancer treatment?
- What long-term side effects may be associated with this cancer treatment?

Support

- What support services are available to me? And to my family?
- Whom should I call with questions or concerns during non-business hours?
- May I contact you or the nurse to talk about additional information I find?
- Who handles health insurance concerns in your office?

Follow-up care

- What follow-up tests will I need? How often will I need them?

As a cancer patient you are a consumer. The decision process regarding who will prescribe and administer your treatment is not that much different from any other major purchase. But the consequences of your decisions are radically different from those involved in buying an automobile, for example.

You have the right, even the responsibility, to ask questions of your doctor just as you would with any consumer purchase. Evaluate those answers more closely than any major purchase you have ever made. Your options and choices for the best treatment will then become clearer.

Cancer survivors are consumer activists. They ask. Become an activist!

An Essential Thing to Do

Obtain answers to the preceding questions today! Record the answers in your Wellness and Recovery Journal. Ask the same questions again at the time you obtain your second opinion.

#4

GET
A
SECOND
OPINION

Obtain a second opinion from a board-certified oncologist, or cancer specialist. This is a critically important step that is not to be overlooked. If at all possible, the second opinion should be completed prior to starting any treatment program.

Whom you consult is also critically important. Second opinions should come from a multidisciplinary team. Typically you will want to speak to a surgeon, a radiation oncologist, and a medical oncologist. Why? Each will look at your case through his or her own training and experience. A radiation oncologist will typically say, "Radiation." A medical oncologist will typically say, "Chemotherapy." Let each of the oncologists know you will be talking to the other specialist. This knowledge alone will act as another checkpoint of control.

Additionally, the second opinion doctors need to be independent of each other as well as not in a working partnership, formal or informal, with the doctor who made the initial diagnosis. Look for different hospital and medical group affiliations. Many people travel to major cancer centers to obtain them. Second opinion consultations are that important.

Do not be fearful that a request for a second opinion might alienate your doctor. Second opinion consultations are standard procedure; your doctor makes such referrals every day. Ask the doctor who made the initial diagnosis, or a member of the staff, for a complete transcript of your medical records. Then take the records with you, or have them sent ahead. I prefer to personally hand the records to the consulting staff. It eliminates the chance of lost pages and delays.

The cost of obtaining at least one second opinion is reimbursed by virtually all insurance programs. Even if you're not covered, get the second opinion. Don't let cost stand in the way of obtaining some of the most important advice of your life.

"I had a second opinion all right," explained Katherine Gerhardt, a fifty-five-year-old insurance office manager and grandmother, describing her experience with breast cancer. "The second opinion came from another surgeon who shared offices with the first. They both said "radical" (mastectomy) was the way to go. And to this day I wonder if I would have been better off with a lumpectomy and radiation."

Katherine's second opinion experience could have been improved in two ways. First, she would have been better served by consulting with an oncologist. These specialists diagnose and treat cancer every working day. They can be expected to have the most up-to-date information on treatment options for each type and stage of cancer. Both surgeons Katherine consulted were general surgeons who dealt with a variety of illnesses, not just cancer.

Second, Katherine would have been better served by consulting with a second opinion doctor not associated with the first. Her surgeons were located in the same building and just down the hall from her family doctor.

These associations are a little-discussed but potentially important issue to patients. Doctors who are friends, office mates, business associates, or in a junior position within a medical practice may find it difficult to challenge the diagnoses or recommended treatment programs of associates. All sorts of relationships exist that may influence decisions. "We were in the middle of renegotiating the lease," said Robert, a young oncologist who rented office space from another oncologist. "We were meeting that very afternoon to discuss rents. I didn't want to offend my landlord when he sent me a patient for a second opinion consultation. So I just agreed with his treatment recommendations."

That experience may seem improbable, but the story is unfortunately true. The best safeguard is to seek second opinions from board-certified oncologists with different specialties, who are affiliated with different practices, at different hospitals, and perhaps even live in different cities.

It puzzles me why so many cancer patients are fearful of asking for a second opinion. When I have inquired, the typical response is, "No one told me to ask," or, "I don't want to offend my doctor."

Obtaining a second opinion in no way implies that the initial diagnosis is incorrect, that the suggested treatment is inappropriate, or that you lack confidence in the physician. On a subject as important as this, you simply deserve to have the benefit of more than one person's thinking. Your second opinion search also puts you in touch with other doctors, giving you options and helping you decide which medical team will actually administer your treatment program.

John was a sixty-two-year-old accountant diagnosed with colon cancer. His primary care doctor suggested John consult with a surgeon. The day John's second set of test results came back from the lab, the surgeon called John, confirmed the initial diagnosis, and said, "I've scheduled you for surgery. Be at the hospital by six-thirty tomorrow morning." Fortunately, John had the courage to say "slow down" and went about obtaining another second opinion consultation from a board-certified medical oncologist.

The second opinion oncologist independently confirmed the initial diagnosis. In fact, he also recommended surgery, just as John was initially advised. John returned to his surgeon only to be greeted with sarcasm: "I told you so. What's the matter? Didn't you trust me?" John walked out of that doctor's office, found another surgeon, and today is in excellent health. The lessons: second opinions are critical. And you do not have to accept intimidation or arrogance.

An Essential Thing to Do

Make your second opinion appointment today. This is one of the most important things you can do. *Do not overlook this step.* Act now! Pick up the phone. Make the appointment.

#5

BECOME AN
E-PATIENT

Turn to the Internet to research your diagnosis, understand all your treatment options, and connect with other patients similarly diagnosed. Here's a handful of the best resources:

Cancer Recovery Foundation. www.cancerrecovery.org. The award-winning resource for integrated cancer care. Helps you mobilize body, mind, and spirit to get well and stay well. Analysis of conventional, complementary, and alternative treatment options. Extensive nutritional guidance. Suggested exercise regimens. Attitude builders. Support, both individual and groups, online and via telephone. Spiritually inclusive.

Oncolink. www.oncolink.edu. The top medically based cancer Website. Managed by the University of Pennsylvania, this site provides clinical information in understandable language. Comprehensive information about all the specific types of cancers, their conventional treatment options, and research news.

National Cancer Institute. www.cancer.gov. If you are the type of patient who wants and needs technical and medically focused information, this is your source. Here you will find extensive cancer statistics plus information on virtually all cancer diagnoses, conventional treatment options, genetics, clinical trials, and ongoing research.

Mayo Clinic. www.mayoclinic.com. The world-famous Mayo Clinic has an excellent Website for both patients and healthcare professionals. Under their "Health Information" tab, click "Diseases and Conditions" followed by "Cancer." The site's information is offered in patient-friendly language.

Cancer Treatment Centers of America. www.cancercenter.com. When it comes to actual treatment, this site gives patients a multitude of options that few others do. I recommend you visit this Website and contact this organization to determine if their services seem right for you.

Dartmouth Atlas of Health Care. www.dartmouthatlas.org. The Dartmouth Atlas Project documents variations in how medical resources are distributed and used in the United States. The project uses Medicare data to provide information and analysis about national, regional, and local markets, as well as hospitals and their affiliated physicians. Use this site to determine where your hospital and physician ranks compared to best-practice standards.

HealthGrades. www.healthgrades.com. This Website rates doctors and hospitals providing today's best transparent, data-driven outcomes to the public. Visit this site to become informed about the healthcare quality your current team delivers as well as understanding provider options in your area.

Breast Cancer Charities of America. www.thebreastcancer charities.org. Cancer Recovery Foundation's affiliate organization devoted to teaching breast cancer prevention to all women and integrated cancer care to those fighting breast cancer.

Rapid online evolution of cancer information has allowed us as informed healthcare consumers to become much more sophisticated in the kinds of information we can access. There is a plethora of cancer information on the Web. I encourage you to spend time on these sites in order to school yourself on your own cancer diagnosis and treatment.

An Essential Thing to Do

Do the research. Hold yourself accountable for gaining a working knowledge of your diagnosis and all your treatment options.

#6

RETHINK
THE
STATISTICS

As you conduct your research into treatment options, you will invariably discover cancer recovery statistics that detail cancer incidence, mortality, and five-year survival rates. Do not let these statistics paralyze you.

Statistics measure populations. They can be interpreted in a great many ways. But statistics do not determine any individual case, including yours.

Let's look squarely at the facts about cancer. According to the National Cancer Institute's SEER (Surveillance Epidemiology and End Results; http://seer.cancer.gov) studies, anyone can develop cancer. However, the risk of being diagnosed increases with age. Nearly 80 percent of cancers are diagnosed in people fifty-five years of age and older. Approximately one in two men and one in three women will be diagnosed with cancer in their lifetime.

Lifestyle choices have an immensely powerful impact on the risk of being diagnosed with cancer. For example, a male smoker's risk of developing lung cancer is approximately twenty-five times greater than that of a nonsmoker. Genetic factors impact only about 5 percent of cancers. For example, a woman whose mother, sister, or daughter had breast cancer is approximately twice as likely to be diagnosed as someone who does not have this family history. These inherited genetics pale in comparison to damaged genetics caused by external factors such as tobacco, alcohol, environmental toxins, and too much exposure to sunlight, as well as internal factors such as overuse of hormones and poor nutrition.

Unfortunately, approximately 1.6 million new cancer diagnoses will be made this year in the United States and approximately 600,000 people will die from cancer. The good news is that nearly 12 million Americans have received a cancer diagnosis and have survived. You can be one of those people.

Your response to these statistics is critical. Realize that statistics measure populations. They can be interpreted in a great many ways. But statistics do not determine any individual case, including yours.

Just after my second surgery, I received a booklet filled with numerical tables, statistics, and graphs on all types of cancers. Of course I felt compelled to read all the information on lung cancer. The numbers on metastatic lung cancer were not promising. As I reflected on what I read, I felt frightened, depressed, and filled with despair, certain of my fast-approaching death.

Several days later I looked again at those statistics and realized that many people do survive. "What did the survivors do?" I wondered. "How can I learn from them?"

No matter how difficult your situation, realize that there is no type of cancer that does not have some rate of survival. This is a significant fact, and it is cause for reasonable hope. The question now becomes, "What can I do to maximize my chances of getting on the right side of these statistics?"

With this book you have already begun to tap into the answers.

An Essential Thing to Do

Interpret statistics as indications of progress. Determine to act with the conviction that you will be counted among the "survivor statistics."

THE SECOND STEP: DETERMINE YOUR TREATMENT

Cancer calls for a rational plan of treatment. After understanding your diagnosis, you will have several treatment options to consider. Much of the conventional treatment recommendations will depend on a combination of the results of your pathology report and the treatment customs in your geographic area.

You have the central role to play in this decision. Your treatment plan needs to balance the physician's recommendations with your beliefs and wishes about what is best for you. This section will help you make a step-by-step evaluation to arrive at the treatment plan that is right for you. Let's move on to this next series of decisions.

#7

UNDERSTAND YOUR CONVENTIONAL TREATMENT OPTIONS

In addition to the information you generate from your own research, you should expect your oncologist to carefully explain which type of conventional treatment(s) is recommended for your type and stage of cancer. The options will typically fall into one or a combination of three primary treatment modalities:

- Surgery: removal of the tumor
- Radiation: exposure to X-rays or radium
- Chemotherapy: the use of cytotoxic chemicals

Surgery is the most frequently employed cancer treatment. It is best used when the cancer is small and has not moved to other parts of the body. Radiation therapy is employed in approximately one-half of all cancer cases. It is often used in combination with other treatment options, for example either before or after surgery. Chemotherapy is most often used when the cancer has spread or when the diagnosis is a systemic-type cancer. It is often used in combination with radiation therapy and surgery to control tumor growth.

Three other types of conventional medical treatment modalities are being used more frequently:

- Hormonal: employs or manipulates bodily hormones
- Immunotherapy: enhancing the body's own immune function
- Investigative: experimental programs

Hormonal treatment is used in cancers that depend on hormones for their growth. Hormones are either removed, added, or their production is blocked through drugs or surgery that removes the hormone-producing gland. Immunotherapy includes the cytokines, like the family of interleukins and interferons, and is an attempt to boost or restore the body's natural defense system. Many people believe immunotherapies will soon comprise a fourth widely accepted treatment modality. At this writing, their scientific efficacy is yet to be established. Investigative protocols are experimental. They are typically the last choice.

As you evaluate your conventional treatment options, please carefully consider some of my personal observations from over two decades of helping patients make informed choices:

1. While surgery is the most common form of conventional treatment, dozens of types of cancer diagnosis do not indicate surgery. Many patients panic when they are told their cancer is "inoperable." If you have been told that your cancer in inoperable, do not despair. Recognize that inoperable does not equate with incurable!

If your oncologist suggests surgery, and you concur, the decision as to who actually performs the procedure is yours. Your choice of surgeons is important. You're more likely to get a well-qualified surgeon if you choose one who is a fellow of the American College of Surgeons and who is also board certified in his or

her field. Only about half of practicing surgeons are board certified, so be sure to ask.

Special note to premenopausal breast cancer patients:

You typically have some flexibility on the timing of your surgery. Scientific evidence is mounting that fewer breast cancer
recurrences are reported among women who choose to have
their surgery during the luteal phase of the menstrual cycle, i.e.,
fourteen to thirty days following the onset of menstruation. Except for one Canadian study that suggested day 8 to be the optimal time, research shows surgery performed in the latter half
of the menstrual cycle results in the fewest recurrences. Ask
your surgeon for the most up-to-date research information prior
to scheduling. You may have to assert yourself here; most surgeries are scheduled at the convenience of the surgeon and/or
the hospital.

2. Thoroughly understand chemotherapy. Before you say yes
to chemotherapy, ask to see proof, such as scientific papers and
reports, on the effectiveness of the treatment being offered. Examine the hard evidence that the suggested chemotherapy protocol actually *cures, extends life, or improves quality of life.* Those
are the three "outcomes" against which you must measure all
treatments—conventional, experimental, complementary, and
alternative.

If your clinician uses the terms "response" or "tumor response"
or "reduce the tumor burden" or "achieve a remission," these
represent different standards. These terms mean shrinkage or
stopping the progression of the cancer. None of these terms are
synonymous with "cure." A cure actually requires that your body
fight the cancer on a cellular level and that your immune system
maintain a disease-free state. To maximize your opportunity for
such a response, I encourage you to follow as many of the health-
enhancing, life-enriching principles in this book as possible.

Study the chemotherapy treatment option in depth. Do your
own research. Ask about both short-term and long-term side ef-

fects. Request the names and phone numbers of long-term survivors who were treated with similar regimens. Ask for their experience and analysis. Know exactly what you can expect—and not expect—chemotherapy to accomplish. Once you possess that information, you are in a position to make a truly informed decision. (See previous section, Caution: Overtreatment, page 43, for a more detailed discussion of chemotherapy options.)

3. Radiation therapy is most often administered by means of an external beam machine. Internal radiation is becoming more common, where radioactive material is surgically implanted into or on the area to be treated. This procedure requires precision. You will maximize your opportunity for receiving excellent care if you choose a physician who is certified by the American Board of Radiology. Ask.

Proton beam therapy is an advanced type of radiation treatment that uses a beam of protons to deliver radiation directly to the tumor, destroying the malignant cells while sparing healthy tissues. Protons enter the body with a low radiation dose, stop at the tumor, match its shape and volume, and deposit the bulk of their cancer-fighting energy right at the tumor.

This new technology is excellent especially for lung cancer, prostate cancer, lymphomas, esophageal cancer, as well as brain and skull base cancers. Although not curative, proton therapy is also used in liver and pancreatic cancer to relieve pain. It can also be used for treatment of soft tissue sarcomas, a relatively rare cancer.

I am particularly encouraged by the rapid advances of proton beam radiation. Because the technology is expensive, it is currently found only at major cancer centers. Go to the National Association for Proton Therapy's Website, www.proton-therapy.org, to find the hospital nearest you.

All cancers are treatable. Even in cases where the cancer is advanced, experimental investigative programs are available. See www.clinicaltrials.gov. If your cancer is not responding to conventional treatment, ask about hormonal treatment and biological response modifiers. Especially consider the many complementary and alternative programs described in this book. You are entitled to understand the full range of treatments available. From that understanding, you will have the knowledge and power to make the most intelligent treatment decisions.

Conventional treatment has its important place. In interviews with and surveys of more than 16,000 cancer survivors, over 96 percent stated they initiated a course of conventional therapy. It is a myth that cancer survivors turn exclusively to alternative, nontraditional cancer treatments in large numbers. In the late 1980s, a Food and Drug Administration study estimated that 40 percent of cancer patients used unconventional treatments. That may be true; in fact, I believe the number may now be much higher, perhaps 75 percent. But survivors do not give up the traditional treatments. They integrate complementary and alternative practices into a comprehensive recovery program. That is what the guidance in this book is all about.

A final thought on conventional treatment options:

Please clearly understand this point: the vast majority of survivors select a conventional program using surgery, chemotherapy, or radiation, often in combination, as the foundation of their treatment. Survivors then supplement this conventional approach with many of the ideas presented in this book. I recommend you implement a conventional medical treatment program based on your own research and your own strong belief. However, I also believe your treatment is not complete until you initiate a comprehensive and integrated cancer recovery program. Given our current levels of understanding, this integration represents your very best opportunity for surviving cancer.

An Essential Thing to Do

Ask your oncologist to explain the specific treatment options available to you in the areas of surgery, radiation, and chemotherapy. Ask also about hormonal, immunotherapy, and investigative programs. Ask for his or her recommendation. Then check these recommendations against the "What to Expect in Treatment" section of the Cancer Recovery Foundation Website, www.cancer recovery.org. Record this information in your Wellness and Recovery Journal. *Do not* give your approval for treatment just yet. First, more work remains to be completed.

#8

GAUGE YOUR CONFIDENCE IN YOUR MEDICAL TEAM

Few patients have any objective way to judge whether their surgeons, oncologists, or other medical professionals have technical competence. We can consider our medical team's education and professional certifications, and the experiences of other patients. But few of us can evaluate, with technical accuracy, whether a particular doctor will be able to address our specific case with success. We can, however, make subjective assessments, the kind of judgments that can be enormously important in our recovery journey. We can intuitively gauge our confidence level.

Ann Simmons, a highly successful insurance executive, was diagnosed with ovarian cancer. By the time it was discovered, the metastasis was significant and the prognosis poor. Ann interviewed seven different oncologists. She went to them with her pathology report and diagnosis in hand and simply asked, "Assuming this diagnosis is correct, what would you have me do?"

The answers she received were actually fairly predictable and consistent. That was reassuring. But what was more comforting was one oncologist's interpersonal skills. He listened. He asked questions to determine Ann's confidence in a procedure. Based on Ann's answers, and her confidence level, he offered his recommendations. Ann chose this doctor.

Ann's analysis was based not so much on any objective measures of technical competence but on her intuition, her belief in a person and a recommended program. She followed that intuition.

I believe you can trust your intuition provided you double-check it. To be sure, an excellent bedside manner can seldom make up for a lack of training, knowledge, and technical expertise. But survivors have repeatedly told me there is a direct correlation between the confidence one has in one's healthcare team and the probability of recovery. Communication skills shape that confidence level. You are seeking a balance here.

An Essential Thing to Do

Evaluate your confidence level following an encounter with members of your medical team. This is particularly important when you are being asked to make treatment decisions. If you harbor more doubt than assurance toward your healthcare providers and their recommendations, it is time to change either your confidence level or your team.

Be sure you are approaching this work at a comfortable pace. I suggest you take a break now and reflect on this important step. Continue your work after you have rested.

#9

CONVICTION VERSUS WISHFUL THINKING

Following an ovarian cancer diagnosis, Elaine Bothwell, a busy mother and community volunteer, was told by her oncologist that an aggressive course of chemotherapy, one that would require hospitalization, was recommended.

Elaine deeply feared chemotherapy. Still vivid in her memory was her mother-in-law's agonizing death from cancer. The side effects of treatment were much worse than the illness. Elaine vowed at that time if she were ever diagnosed with cancer she would never have chemotherapy. Now she faced precisely the situation she feared most.

Elaine went in search of nontraditional treatments. Among others, she consulted a naturopath who suggested metabolic therapy, a combination of detoxification, herbs, and hyperthermia (the use of heat) to help destroy cancer cells. While this program sounded minimally toxic and noninvasive, Elaine now feared she was getting too far away from conventional medical care.

Then Elaine went to another medical oncologist. After she explained her fears and her search, this doctor recommended the use of hormones. Elaine was assured that hormonal therapy was typically less toxic than chemotherapy and in most cases generated far fewer side effects. But the hormone treatment was not as highly recommended as the original and more effective chemotherapy program.

Torn between these three different approaches, Elaine realized that the treatment she was most convinced would work was a combination of two. Through sheer persistence she was able to find a cancer treatment center that combined fractionated-dose chemotherapy with hyperthermia. On her own, she adopted a nutritional supplementation program that included the herbs. She decided to hold the hormone treatment in reserve.

Elaine's choice of treatment is clearly not the answer for everyone. But following one's conviction is an important element of nearly every successful treatment program. Today, twenty-four years after her initial diagnosis, Elaine's cancer remains in remission, and she leads a full and happy life.

"I wanted conviction from my doctor," said Bill Follett, a colon cancer survivor. "I looked him right in the eyes and asked, 'Is this treatment just the conventional thinking, Doctor? Or can you show me the hard data to back up your recommendation?' When he reviewed the published research, it seemed surgery followed by chemotherapy was my best bet."

An Essential Thing to Do

Before you commit to a treatment program, take the time to ask yourself some critical questions: "Do I hold the belief that this is the right thing to be doing?" "Am I just taking the path of least resistance?" If you don't believe in it, resist! Find a treatment program that you can follow with conviction.

#10

REFLECT ON THE TREATMENT DECISION

If you've carefully read each step up to this point, you'll realize that you've simply been gathering information about treatment options. You have not yet made any treatment decisions. Now it is time to systematically review your treatment options one last time prior to crossing this Rubicon.

First, compare. Are you receiving consistent information from:

- The doctor who made the initial diagnosis?
- The oncologists whom you consulted for your second opinion?
- The recommendations you found through your independent research?

You should expect to see a reasonable consistency in the recommendations you receive from these sources. Most treatment variances should relate to differences in levels of toxicity and degrees of invasiveness. If there is fundamental agreement, your decision-making process will probably be straightforward.

If the recommendations are inconsistent, then your information gathering is not complete. When you receive mixed signals, it is a certain sign to obtain another qualified and independent opinion. This is time and money wisely spent.

Several providers in the oncology community have criticized me for this suggestion. Their objections have included: "The differences in treatment that you'll find are actually very minor." "Most patients cannot afford the cost." "You're just losing valuable time in receiving treatment." I disagree.

In all but the very rare case, the few days spent in gaining third or fourth opinions are well worth the wait. We can all find the funds if necessary. As a patient you are after the very best treatment. You should expect a consistency of recommendations, if not a consensus.

Terry Bartholomew is a forty-seven-year-old man from Indiana who was diagnosed with lymphoma. He obtained eight different opinions before agreeing to a program of treatment. Terry's determination to find the best has proven wise, and today he is alive and well.

Terry's experience points to an objection patients often raise: "But my insurance won't cover a third or fourth opinion." My response is, "Find a way." I was only too glad to pay for the services of qualified medical experts who would help determine the best course of treatment for me. Develop a similar attitude. Don't let insurance coverage limits determine this issue. Borrow the money or even seek out a free clinic. There is nothing more important in your life at this moment.

Once you attain clarity and conviction in terms of the medical treatment, another evaluation needs a second reflective look. Are you comfortable with the people who will give you treatment and the place where the treatment will be administered?

June Callas, a single mother in her fifties, had ovarian cancer. The treatment program in which she had the most confidence was recommended by doctors at a cancer center that was located more than an hour's commute over busy California freeways. She was expected to visit the center weekly while undergoing treatment. The commute was a problem. June didn't want to drive in rush-hour traffic; a friend or family member would have to act as chauffeur. She also didn't feel completely safe in the part of the city where the treatment center was located.

June expressed her concerns about the drive and her physical safety to the supervising oncologist. The doctor's response was compassionate and understanding. He was able to make arrangements at a hospital only ten minutes from June's apartment. She could receive her weekly treatments there and visit the cancer center just once a month. To this day, June believes the change in location was an important part of her successful recovery.

Does the recommended treatment program truly have your conviction? Are you convinced that the recommendations are the finest? Conviction implies a sense of certainty. While there are no guarantees, your treatment program and the people who administer it should elicit a strong degree of certainty that this is the right path to be taking at this time.

Cancer Recovery Foundation has helped thousands of cancer patients walk through this treatment option analysis. Invariably a question arises: "What about all the alternative approaches? I really haven't checked them out." We have consistently recommended this strategy: First, explore the conventional treatment options. Surgery, radiation, and chemotherapy are the basis for the overwhelming majority of survivor success stories.

If the conventional treatment methods hold no real promise, then analyze both the investigative options as well as the complementary and alternative therapies.

With all the options, integrate improved diet and nutritional supplementation, gentle exercise plus the psychosocial and psychospiritual techniques. Mobilize body, mind, and spirit. I believe that a physician who withholds this integrated treatment approach is no longer offering an informed medical opinion.

Allow yourself time to reflect on these important decisions. Don't be pressured by anyone to hurry a decision. When the treatment recommendations are consistent, the people who administer the treatment have your confidence; you understand the importance of integrating body, mind, and spirit; and you can say with conviction that this is what you should be doing now. Then, and only then, are you ready to go to the next step.

An Essential Thing to Do

Consult your notations in your Wellness and Recovery Journal. Thoughtfully, carefully, systematically, reflect on your treatment decision. Take another break. Reflect . . . again.

#11

DECIDE!

There is power in decision.

The cancer journey is made up of both little decisions and big decisions. Your treatment program is a big one. In many ways it will determine the direction of your entire life. Now is the time to decide.

Decision is the spark that ignites action. Until a decision is reached, nothing happens.

Making decisions like this takes courage. But there is power in facing the fact that you have cancer, then carefully doing your homework, and finally choosing a course of action. Without exercising your courage, the problem will remain forever unaddressed.

Decide! Do not straddle the fence or make a partial decision. This is the time to take a firm stand on one side or another. Make a full commitment.

Yes, you will monitor your decision. You will keep your options open, of course. But now is the moment to say, "This is how we will climb the mountain! Now let's get started!"

Decision frees us from many of the uncertainties caused by

fear, doubt, and anxiety. Yes, there is risk. But there is greater risk in making no decision, hoping that all will magically be well.

Decide. You've done the work. This is not blind chance. This decision is the culmination of careful and sustained inquiry. Now is the time for action.

Decision awakens the spirit. Do you feel a new awakening? Do you sense that part of you is springing to life? Nourish that spirit. Cherish it. It is the life force inside you working for you, helping you get well again.

Decide. The decision comes first, the results follow. Today is the day. Now is the hour. This is the moment! Decide!

An Essential Thing to Do

Now, make the treatment decision. Appreciate the power of your commitment. Be optimistic. Decide! Inform your team of your choice.

#12

GIVE ONLY INFORMED CONSENT

All treatment decisions should be made—must be made—with the informed consent of the patient or patient's guardian. This means you need to know in detail, in terms you can clearly understand, all the risks entailed in any procedure involving surgery, anesthesia, radiation therapy, chemotherapy, or a similar medical procedure.

You'll be asked to sign a consent form. Do not sign a blank consent form. Make certain that the exact procedure is described and that you fully understand it. You have the right to set limits on these documents. You can cross out statements to which you do not consent. For example, I drew a line through the section of my consent form that asked my permission to videotape the operation for the removal of my lung.

You have the right to refuse treatment. An adult who is mentally competent can refuse treatment even if it may result in death. Nancy was a young woman who was pregnant. Even though she was advised to go ahead with treatment for lung cancer, she felt so strongly about the potential harm to her unborn child that she elected to postpone treatment until after her delivery. She exercised her right to refuse consent.

You need to understand clearly and completely all to which you are consenting. Gary Nadine, a retired pilot who made his home in Oregon, recognized that something was wrong with his health when he began to feel weak all the time. In six months he lost more than twenty pounds without dieting. "I just wasn't hungry," he said. "And I felt like I had a low-grade fever all the time." Then Gary became aware of swelling in his abdomen.

Finally he went to his doctor, who ordered a variety of tests. There was a complete physical examination, the most thorough he had ever experienced. Then chest X-rays, CAT scans, a blood workup, urine tests, and more. After consulting with other specialists, the doctor finally told Gary he had Hodgkin's disease.

Gary signed a consent form that said "laparotomy," thinking that he was giving permission for a biopsy. "The way it was presented," said Gary, "this seemed like just another test to determine, with more certainty, the extent of the disease. The doctor told me they needed to know where the cancer had spread. I thought it was no big deal and that I'd be out of the hospital the next day."

In fact, it was a big deal and Gary was not fully informed. A laparotomy is a surgical procedure that allows the doctors to explore the entire abdominal area. It is major surgery that should only be done by a team of experienced surgeons. Because of complications and infections, Gary's hospital stay lasted two and a half weeks. It left him with significant scars and lasting discomfort.

While Gary technically, even legally, gave consent to the procedure, in his mind he gave his okay for something much different. "I should have asked," lamented Gary. "But it seemed like no big deal."

Your doctor is obligated to inform you fully of any procedure to which you are being asked to give consent. This means explaining to you the procedure's purpose and risks, other alternatives, and the risk involved in not having the procedure. Don't be intimidated by the medical lingo. Make certain you get this information in language you understand. More important, make certain you ask detailed questions prior to giving any consent. Don't tolerate a physician's attitude that your concerns are unwelcome. If he or she is condescending or overly impatient, find another doctor. And be certain to include on your list of questions, "Why is this procedure absolutely necessary?"

An Essential Thing to Do

Ask your physician—not an associate, not an assistant, and not a nurse—to describe clearly the risks involved in your tests and treatment. Compare the risks to the expected benefits.

THE THIRD STEP: MANAGE YOUR TREATMENT

The cancer journey can be a winding road, a complex navigational task. Ultimately, you the patient are the one who needs to be in charge. Many aspects come into play, including all the medical appointments, medical tests, and, most important, your self-care.

All of these matters are your responsibility to monitor and implement. But the effort is manageable. Let's explore some simple but powerful ideas that will make treatment management easier.

#13

BELIEVE
IN YOUR
TREATMENT
PROGRAM

Excited belief is one of the great intangibles in a successful cancer treatment program. It is a natural extension of your conviction about your integrated treatment decisions. And it is your personal responsibility to believe in, and even be excited about, your treatment program.

Rachael Katz and May Tyson both attended one of our Cancer Recovery seminars in Atlanta. Rachael is a Georgia homemaker who started a course of radiation following surgery for breast cancer. Her attitude toward treatment was, "I guess it's something I have to do."

May received virtually the same diagnosis about a month after Rachael. May also had surgery and a follow-up course of chemotherapy. But her attitude was totally different from Rachael's: "I saw those chemicals as a great healing agent, something coming into my body to make me well. I welcomed my chemotherapy with open arms!"

Today May is free of cancer. Rachael continues to struggle.

Cancer survivors develop a confidence and an *excited belief* in their treatment programs that other patients do not possess. I am convinced that a direct correlation exists between belief in one's treatment and its effectiveness. My observations of the importance of belief in cancer treatment lead me to respect the awesome power of the mind and the human spirit in the cancer journey. I want to see you mobilize those resources in your own program.

Cassandra Pooley is a California wife, mother, and now retired elementary school teacher. After three years of remission, she had a recurrence of breast cancer including liver and bone metastasis. Her doctors gave her less than a year to live. "I knew I was at the crossroads," said Cassandra. "And when I learned that survivors held an excited belief about their treatment, I knew I had to change my expectations and get excited."

You can observe excited and expectant belief in survivor after survivor. I fully realize my observations are only anecdotal evidence and cannot stand up to scientific scrutiny. But I do believe this hypothesis is true. Cancer survival is a matter of involving both head and heart. I have seen beliefs and attitudes like May's and Cassandra's make the difference in hundreds of cases. To me the correlation between belief in treatment and effectiveness of treatment is very high.

Someday the scientific and medical communities will fully document the biological reality of this kind of optimism. In the meantime, I suggest you not enter the debate. Instead, learn from the survivors and develop an excited belief about your treatment.

An Essential Thing to Do

"Own" your treatment program. See it as a friend. Believe it is there to help you. Excited belief is what you seek.

#14

Overcome Fatigue and Nausea

Extreme fatigue is reported by nearly 90 percent of cancer patients both during and after treatment. Worse, getting more sleep or rest often does not relieve the fatigue. In fact, cancer-related fatigue is one of the most profound and distressing survival issues patients face. This unique type of fatigue can have dozens of causes, and for patients who have completed cancer therapy, fatigue is among their foremost concerns, second only to fear of disease recurrence.

What can be done? Moderate exercise is the number one treatment for fatigue. In patient after patient, exercise was found to mitigate fatigue and lead to more restful and predictable sleep. You'll find more information on this important thing to do in section 26 of this book.

In addition, the popular dietary supplement ginseng appears to relieve fatigue and boost energy levels in people with cancer. Researchers studied 282 people with breast, colon, and other types of cancer. They were randomly assigned to take 750 milligrams, 1,000 milligrams, or 2,000 milligrams of American ginseng or a placebo daily for eight weeks.

About 25 percent of those on the two highest doses reported their fatigue was "moderately or much better," compared with only 10 percent of those taking the lowest dose or the placebo. Also, energy levels were about twice as high in those taking the 1,000-milligram dose as those taking the placebo.

People taking the two highest doses also reported generally feeling better, with improvements in mental, physical, spiritual, and emotional well-being. And they said they were more satisfied with their treatment.

The researchers tested the Wisconsin species of American ginseng, which is different from Chinese ginseng and other forms of American ginseng sold in health food stores. The ginseng was powdered and given in capsule form. However, the question remains unanswered on interactions with some conventional medical treatments.

Next is nausea. One of the realities for about half of the cancer patients undergoing chemotherapy is nausea. While there are other side effects, including hair loss, fatigue, and the decreased ability of the body to make red and white blood cells and platelets, nausea is typically the most uncomfortable. It may or may not include vomiting. Most people can significantly improve this experience, but it takes some experimentation. Here are some suggestions:

- Ask your oncologist for antinausea medication. Compazine, Tigan, and Zofran are commonly prescribed. Try taking them thirty to sixty minutes before treatments.
- Use relaxation exercises. (See section 34.)
- Eat smaller meals more often. Try six daily meals.
- Emphasize low-fat foods, especially fresh fruits.
- Limit liquids taken with meals. Drink no liquids in the hour before meals and the hour following meals. But be sure to take in enough liquids at other times. If you choose chemotherapy, your oncologist will tell you to drink more liquids to ensure good urine flow and minimize problems with the liver, kidneys, and bladder.

- Clear, cool liquids are recommended. Iced green tea, ginger ale, clear broths, ice pops, or apple juice ice cubes are worth trying. Take all liquids slowly.
- Eat dry food such as crackers, toast, or popcorn—especially at the start of the day or at the first sign of nausea. Sorry, no butter on the popcorn.
- Do not lie down for two hours after eating. You can rest sitting up. Or if you simply must stretch out, prop a couple of pillows under your head to gain elevation.
- Sometimes loose clothing or fresh air will help in nausea control.
- Ask your pharmacist about Travel-Eze or Seaband antinausea wrist bands.
- Drink ginger root tea steeped with peppermint.
- Goldenseal root may be helpful.
- Try hypnosis. Several small clinical trials have shown significant reductions in nausea and vomiting versus no hypnotherapy.

An Essential Thing to Do

Experiment. Clearly, there is no one-size-fits-all answer to fatigue and nausea. You'll need to try the suggested ideas. They have proven successful for many other cancer patients. They may be just the answer you have been searching for.

#15

Make the Most of Your Appointments

Free and open communication between you and your healthcare team is one of the most important aspects of your cancer recovery journey. You need to stay informed. You want feedback. But seldom is this information volunteered. You'll have to ask for it.

Wise patients bring a list of questions to virtually every medical appointment. If you have continuing or new symptoms, ask about them. If you are experiencing side effects, ask about them. Ask for further information about issues raised from your reading or from talking to other patients.

"My radiation technician started to tease me about all my questions," said a retired Minneapolis professor who was being treated for prostate cancer. "I'd walk in the room and she'd say, 'What's on your list today, Dr. Nelson?' But I was determined to participate fully, to be an active patient. So I didn't let her remarks bother me in the least."

Speak with total honesty to your doctor and the entire healthcare team. They are not mind readers. Tell them your problems and ask for their opinions. Bring a family member with you if you have trouble being assertive. He or she can be your advocate. Many people are intimidated by their doctors. If you are one of these people, recognize it and act immediately to remove that needless hurdle. If you are having trouble understanding and absorbing medical information, bring a tape recorder. Then you'll be able to review explanations and instructions at your convenience.

In case this hasn't been emphasized enough by now, please understand that your ability to ask questions is one of your most significant points of power. When in doubt, write down your questions and then read them from your list.

One other insider's tip: if you truly want to make the most of your medical appointments, get in the habit of expressing your sincere gratitude to your medical team. One of a group of doctors at a large healthcare system in Pittsburgh lamented to me, "We try so earnestly to help a patient. I wish once in a while they would simply say thank you." I clearly remember giving an appreciative hug to my oncologist. From that day forward I was treated like royalty in that office. Start showing your appreciation to these very important people in your life. Remember, they're people who respond to you just as you respond to them.

An Essential Thing to Do

In your Wellness and Recovery Journal, record both your medical questions and the answers you are given. Keep this information handy. Bring it to your appointments. If you rely on your memory or record your questions on bits of paper scattered here and there, you'll never obtain timely and accurate information.

Write a thank-you note to at least one person on your medical team following your next visit.

#16

MONITOR
YOUR
PROGRESS

As you continue your treatment program, you'll be given tests to determine how well it's working. Ask about the tests prior to agreeing to them. Then insist that the doctor share the results in the form of copies of your test reports.

It's uplifting to know that you are making progress. But even a report that is less encouraging can have a positive side. It should lead you to consider other forms of treatment. Many exist. If all standard therapies have been exhausted, ask about investigative treatments. Or look more seriously at the complementary and alternative choices.

It is your responsibility to monitor your treatment program. Don't wait. Ask.

An Essential Thing to Do

Ask your doctor how and when he or she will check the progress of your treatment. Write this information in your Wellness and Recovery Journal. Then be certain tests occur as scheduled.

The Fourth Step:
Heal
Your
Lifestyle

I am frequently asked, "How much did conventional medicine contribute to your survival?" My answer has been the same for over a decade: 10–15 percent. In my estimation, personal lifestyle choices were absolutely the key reason I am alive today.

A Stanford University health newsletter estimated that lifestyle issues such as poor diet, lack of exercise, and unwise health habits accounted for 61 percent of premature deaths due to cancer. They estimated the proportional share of genetics was 29 percent, and medical treatments themselves were listed as contributing to 10 percent of cancer deaths. I believe these estimates are probably low.

The central point is obvious: lifestyle choices are critical in the cancer survival journey. These are under our control, a matter of intention, an issue of personal choice. Clearly, there is much we can do to help ourselves get well and stay well. Let's examine how literally millions of people have helped in their own healing.

#17

LIVE "WELL"

Make wellness a way of life. Wellness is a stance one chooses in order to maximize one's health—physically, emotionally, and spiritually. The goal is to achieve the highest level of well-being possible in each of these areas of life.

Wellness recognizes and acts on the fact that everything one thinks, says, does, feels, and believes has an impact on one's well-being.

Wellness can be chosen at any moment, in any circumstance. Wellness is possible with disability, regardless of physical condition.

For most people, "living well" typically means some major changes in lifestyle—in body, mind, and spirit.

We previously stated that cancer survivorship is a combination of head and heart. Conquering cancer demands that you reach beyond the physical issues of illness. Your mental, emotional, and spiritual health has a powerful effect on your well-being.

Kelly Liddle is a forty-eight-year-old account executive with a major investment management firm. He developed malignant melanoma. "I went through the surgery and radiation just as recommended," said Kelly. "But I knew the real problem. I wasn't taking care of myself." Kelly hadn't exercised for years. His diet and nutrition habits were deplorable. He despised his work, and his marriage was coming apart.

Like so many survivors, Kelly considered cancer his wake-up call. "I realized my life was off course. And I knew it was up to me to change."

Similar sentiments are expressed by many survivors of cancer. They see illness as a message to make life changes. Kelly went on to reflect, "When I quit my job and opened a floral shop, my entire life started to heal. Cancer has actually been very good for me."

Living well, intentional choice, exercising the decision to take personal responsibility for one's total well-being—this is common talk among cancer survivors. It's whole-person wellness, a triumphant way of living without conditions.

Without conditions means that although wellness may be obscured by illness, it is a matter of personal choice whether wellness will be destroyed by illness. *Without conditions* means it is possible to discover high-level emotional and spiritual wellness in the very midst of life-threatening illness. The decision to "live well" is significant and profound. Never again will your well-being be a static state measured simply by the lack of negative physical symptoms.

My friend, I want to help you catch this vision for your health and your life. Join me. Let's make wellness our shared personal quest.

An Essential Thing to Do

Begin the wellness quest. Open your mind and spirit to whole-person wellness. In your Wellness and Recovery Journal, record one step you can take today to improve your greater well-being. Now act, doing what is clearly doable today. Determine to live life at a new and higher level of wellness no matter what.

#18

OPERATE UNDER NEW ASSUMPTIONS

Compare the assumptions behind orthodox healthcare with those behind whole-person wellness:

Assumptions behind conventional healthcare	Assumptions behind whole-person wellness
1. The patient is reliant upon the medical community.	1. The patient has, or should develop, independence.
2. The professional is the authority.	2. The professional is a healing partner.
3. Symptoms are treated, not investigated.	3. The underlying causes are sought, plus the symptoms are treated.
4. Specialized and concerned with body's subsystems.	4. Unified and concerned with person's whole life.
5. Body viewed as a series of mechanical functions.	5. Body viewed as a changing system.

6. Primary repairs made with surgery or drugs.

6. Intervention is minimal and appropriate. Noninvasive therapies are used when possible.

7. Pain and illness are purely negative.

7. Pain and illness are messages to value and act upon.

8. Mind and emotions are a secondary factor in health.

8. Mind and emotions are a major factor in health.

9. Body and mind are separate. Spirit has no health impact.

9. Body, mind, and spirit form one unit and always affect each other.

10. Disease prevention is largely environmental: not smoking, attention to diet, exercise, and rest.

10. Wellness means prevention plus wholeness: harmony in relationships, work, goals; a balance of body, mind, and spirit.

There is an important issue behind these assumptions. Your medical team will be helpful in addressing just one part of your cancer journey, the physical disease portion. Wellness encompasses far more. Whole-person well-being is our goal, and the responsibility for achieving it falls to each of us personally.

An Essential Thing to Do

Review the above assumptions. Circle those you believe to be true. Are you a traditionalist? Do you identify with the spirit of whole-person wellness? What does this analysis tell you to do differently? Which assumptions serve you best?

#19

Schedule Your Wellness

All important tasks demand a schedule. And there is no more important work in your life right now than the work of getting well again.

The trouble is, most people keep putting off the work of wellness, thinking they will get to it later. And guess what? They seldom, if ever, get around to it. Or if they do, it's only after everything else that is "important" has been accomplished.

Develop the attitude that there is nothing more important in your life right now than your work of wellness. For the time being, your wellness efforts need to take priority over family, job, community or religious activities, and social obligations. Getting well is your new top priority; you need to incorporate the disciplines of wellness into your daily life.

I actually blocked out my week on a day planner. My typical weekday schedule looked like this while I was in the middle of recovery:

6:00 AM	Wake up
6:15	Exercise
6:45	Meditate
7:00	Shower, eat, and commute
9:00	Work
Noon	Lunch and meditate
1:00 PM	Work
4:30	Commute
5:30	Meditate
6:00	Dinner
7:00	Family time
9:00	Read and meditate
10:00	Sleep

Doctors' appointments were worked in as needed. During commutes I virtually always listened to wellness CDs. Weekends found me devoting even more time to study and meditation. Throughout the entire process, I became gentler with myself, demanding less in the way of outside activities and more in the way of self-care. I took control of my schedule and made the work of wellness my top priority.

An Essential Thing to Do

Start a new page in your Wellness and Recovery Journal. Plan a schedule for your week similar to mine. Minimize obligations that cause undue stress. Give ample "core time" to the wellness disciplines discussed in this book.

After completing your schedule, I suggest you take a break from your wellness work. Start the next section tomorrow or after you have rested. In the meantime, give careful consideration to how you spend your time. Do you understand I am asking you to make wellness a way of life? For most people, this means a major lifestyle shift. Look within. Consider the evidence and the implications of these suggestions. Begin now to modify your schedule to meet your new wellness priorities.

#20

ELIMINATE ACTIVE AND PASSIVE SMOKING

It totally mystifies me how some cancer patients can continue to use tobacco. John Everest had colon cancer. Following surgery, he started a course of chemotherapy. But do you think he quit smoking? No! "I don't have lung cancer," he'd say as he left our Cancer Recovery support sessions.

If I could communicate this any more strongly I would. Stop smoking! If you are a user, cut out any and all tobacco immediately. Cigarettes, cigars, chewing tobacco—all must go. There is no excuse, even nicotine addiction, that is sufficient to continue this harmful habit. Be clear: tobacco is putting cancer-causing chemicals into your body, something you do not need now or ever.

A family practitioner recently shared with me that he was not going to tell his patients to stop smoking. I was stunned and said, "What!?!?" "Some of them enjoy a cigarette," he said. "And besides, I don't want to offend them." My response was that smokers know they should quit, most want to quit and, far from being offended, they want their doctor to help them quit.

If you smoke, stop! The question is not whether you can quit. The question is whether you will quit. I know this firsthand. I started smoking when I was in my teens. There is no doubt that smoking directly contributed to my lung cancer just over twenty years later. In those twenty years I seriously tried to quit five or six times. Willpower alone didn't get the job done. A change in thinking did.

It started with changing my self-perception. I first went from perceiving myself as a smoker to seeing myself as a person who mistakenly chose the behavior of smoking. Seeing smoking as a behavior helped me detach emotionally and psychologically from the cigarettes. I began to perceive myself as a nonsmoker. A change in self-perception can work for you, too.

In addition to never smoking again, eliminate your exposure to passive smoking. A Finnish study revealed up to a one-third drop in circulating levels of vitamin C and other antioxidants after just thirty minutes of exposure to secondhand smoke.

It has never been more important for you to maximize your health. Tobacco use and exposure to secondhand smoke have no place in the quest for wellness.

An Essential Thing to Do

Envision yourself as completely tobacco-free. Wean yourself with a nicotine patch if you must. But develop a self-image of being a nonsmoker deep in your spirit. And stay far, far away from tobacco users while they are smoking.

#21

ADOPT THIS NUTRITIONAL STRATEGY DURING TREATMENT

I was on the phone speaking to a man with metastatic prostate cancer. The subject quickly turned to nutrition. "What about your diet?" I asked. His reply was, "My doctor says I can eat anything I want."

No, dear friend, that may have been a medical opinion. But that was not an informed medical opinion. The days of "eat anything you want" are long behind. In fact, that philosophy may have contributed to the onset of this man's prostate cancer. It certainly detracts from maximizing one's total health and well-being.

Allow me some very straight talk: if you are determined to choose "eat anything" as your nutritional strategy, close this book now. This integrated cancer care program is not for you.

The field of nutritional science is notorious for its lack of definitive answers. As nutritionists will be only too glad to tell you, more research must be done. But there is a great deal we do know about nutrition and its links to our health. In nearly thirty years of work in this field, I have learned two important principles, things you need to know about the link between diet and cancer, two issues that are not in contention among the nutritional gurus. They are:

Fact 1: The Western diet invariably results in the Western diseases.

The Western diet is typically defined as a diet that is comprised of lots of processed foods and meats, and contains significant amounts of added sugars, fats, salts, and preservatives plus lots of refined grains. This diet minimizes or leaves out fresh vegetables, fresh fruits, and whole grains.

The inevitable result of this Western diet is that the population suffers from high rates of obesity, diabetes, cardiovascular disease, and cancer. Credible research indicates nearly all of the obesity and type 2 diabetes, over 80 percent of the cardiovascular diseases, and at least half of cancers in the United States are linked to this diet. Sound familiar?

Fact 2: People who eat more natural diets suffer far less from the Western diseases.

While there is no single diet that can be prescribed for disease prevention and recovery, this much is clear. Those who eat minimal amounts of trans fats, maintain a high ratio of polyunsaturated to saturated fats, enjoy six or more servings of fresh vegetables and fruits per day, consume high amounts of whole grains, and have two or three servings of fish per week have lower rates of the Western diseases.

The hopeful fact is that people who switch from the Western diet to the natural diet see significant improvements in health. In the process, they help prevent and even reverse the typical Western diseases.

In the Road Map to Recovery section of this book, we briefly discussed nutritional strategy. Let's review. The most common nutritional shifts employed by cancer survivors are the following:

- Whole foods
- Foods low in fat, salt, and sugar
- Fresh vegetables, fresh fruits, and whole grains
- Adequate amounts of pure water

The single major dietary shift among cancer survivors is consuming foods that are less processed. If it is boxed or bottled or canned or packaged, the food comes under immediate scrutiny. Prepared foods, even when enriched, tend to deliver calories with less nutrition than their fresh counterparts. This means cancer survivors spend most of their grocery shopping time in the produce section of their local market.

Whole food means:

Fresh vegetables, fresh fruits, whole grains, whole grain pastas, brown rice, raw nuts, sprouted breads, and the like. See the cancer recovery shopping list in the next section.

Low fat, salt, and sugar means:

Good fats, like unsaturated fats, often classified into two groups: the omega-3s and the omega-6s. They come from extra virgin olive oil, sesame oil, seeds—especially flaxseed—and fatty fish.

Low salt means the right salt—sea salt or liquid aminos.

Low sugar means no added sugar. Sugar should come exclusively from whole food sources and then only in moderation.

Furthermore, please hear me on the importance of avoiding refined sugar. Scientists call sugar an "obligate glucose metabolizer." Loosely translated that means a "feeder." There exists significant evidence-based research pointing to sugar as doing two things that stand in the way of cancer recovery. First, sugar suppresses immune function. Second, it feeds cancer cells.

Diets high in sugar, and foods that turn into sugar when digested, cause blood sugar levels to rise. Once this spike is triggered, the body releases a hormone called insulin in an effort to bring the blood sugar levels back to normal. Understand this next key point: one of insulin's multiple functions is to promote cell growth—be that normal healthy cells or malignant cells. Therefore, the more insulin circulating in the body, the more opportunity for cancer cells to be fed, grow, and divide. See Guide 1: Cancer and Sugar for a more complete discussion of this issue.

So, what can we actually do? Here's your new dietary guideline: "Whites out. Colors in."

"Whites out" mean no:

- White sugar
- White potatoes
- White rice
- White bread
- White pasta

All of these are simple carbohydrates that turn directly into sugar once ingested. Whites out! The days of a couple of teaspoons of sugar into your coffee or even raw or brown sugar onto your cereal are over. Stop eating refined sugar.

"Colors in" means to add:

Fresh vegetables of many colors including broccoli, kale, parsley, cabbage, romaine and leaf lettuce, spinach, peppers, cauliflower, beets, leeks, sweet potatoes, and more.

Fresh fruits of many colors including tomatoes (they are a fruit), apples, lemons, grapes, blueberries, and more. Just consume fruits in lesser quantities than vegetables. The sugar content in fruit is comparatively high.

There has never been a more important time in your life to eat well. Eating whole foods and those low in fat, salt, and sugar while emphasizing fresh fruits and vegetables is your new nutritional program.

An Essential Thing to Do

Wise nutrition is not a problem, it's a decision. So decide. Decide to eat healthfully, better than ever before in your entire life. See nutrition as of utmost importance, equal to or even more important than your medical treatment. Eating right starts with your decision. Decide!

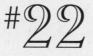

#22

SHOP FOR NUTRIENT-DENSE FOODS

The purpose of this section is to communicate in a clear, practical, and useful manner the best food choices. The best way I know how to do this is by giving you a shopping list. All nutritional education is useless unless and until it is applied. A shopping list is a very good way to apply this knowledge.

The foods on this shopping list "pass the test." A passing grade is based on an analysis of a food's nutrient density. Nutrient density is a factor of vitamin, mineral, protein, fiber, and healthy fat(s) content, plus glycemic index and calories.

Shop from this "Real Foods" list:

Vegetables

___Broccoli*
___Cabbage
___Peppers
___Tomatoes
___Carrots

Fruits

___Berries*
___Oranges
___Red grapefruit
___Mangoes
___Apples

Vegetables

___Leaf lettuce
___Cauliflower
___Onions
___Beets
___Asparagus
___Squash
___Pumpkin

Fruits

___Cherries
___Apricots
___Cantaloupe
___Kiwis*
___Pears
___Red grapes
___Watermelon

Fish, Meat & Eggs

___Cod/flounder/haddock
___Tilapia/Mahi-mahi
___Salmon (wild)*
___Tuna (canned/steaks)
___Trout (wild)
___Shrimp/Blue crab
___Sardines
___Eggs*
___Skinless chicken breast
___Turkey breast

Whole Grains & Breads

___Oats
___Barley
___Brown rice
___Flaxseed
___Buckwheat
___Spelt wheat
___Millet
___Amaranth
___Quinoa
___Wheat germ

Legumes

___Black beans*
___Garbanzo beans
___Kidney beans
___Navy beans
___Pinto beans
___Lentils
___Split peas

Other

___Garlic
___Ginger
___Cinnamon
___Cayenne
___Stevia
___Green tea
___Curry powder

Non-fat Dairy

___Yogurt (plain)*
___Cottage cheese
___Soy milk

Oils

___Extra virgin olive oil
___Sesame oil
___Non-fat vegetable spray

*Superfood: Two servings per week.

On the opposite end of the spectrum, there are several foods that clearly do not receive a passing grade. They deliver calories with few nutrients. This is the "No-Shop" list. During the cancer journey, do not put these foods in your shopping cart.

___Sugar	___Liquor
___Aspartame	___Beer
___Syrups	___Wine
___Hydrogenated fats	___Soft drinks, regular
___Lard	___Soft drinks, diet
___Margarine	___Ice cream
___Salami	___Cookies
___Hot dogs	___Doughnuts
___Bologna	___Cake
___Sausage	___Boxed cereal
___Bacon	___Molasses
___Smoked ham	___Mayonaise
___Pizza	___Honey

This does not mean you can never have another piece of pizza in your life. It does mean that this is the time in your life to "eat clean," meaning whole foods that are nutrient-dense and low in fat, salt, and sugar, with the clear emphasis on fresh vegetables, fresh fruits, and whole grains.

The good news is that there is an endless combination of menus based on nutrient-dense foods. So be creative. Experiment with your menus. You will be contributing to your health and well-being in a major way.

An Essential Thing to Do

If you are in the middle of the cancer journey, hold yourself accountable for shopping and eating from the approved list. See Guide 1: Nutrition as Medicine for a "Real Foods" shopping list you can copy and take to the store.

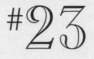

HYDRATE

Adequate pure water means six to eight glasses per day. Hopefully this is non-chlorinated pure spring water. But even tap water is better than being dehydrated.

Water is the basis of all bodily fluids, including digestive fluids, urine, lymph, and perspiration, as well as lubrication of our joints. Water is also essential for all cell activity, especially the transport of waste away from the cells and transport of nutrients to the cells.

Drink water. Coffee, tea, milk, soda, or alcoholic beverages do not count. Water. Pure water is the drink of choice.

It is an almost universal truth—people with cancer are dehydrated. Lack of water inhibits immune function, the most potent defense you have against cancer. The environment your cells live in is not blood, it is fluid. The lymph system, a key component of your immune system, is a fluid system requiring adequate water to function at its highest capacity.

Through natural elimination, perspiration, and even breathing, your body loses water daily. Fluid must be continually replaced in appropriate quantities for you to be optimally well.

I prefer water with no chlorine or fluorides. This is difficult to obtain from most municipal water systems. Even bottled water, especially if contained in plastic, is not a sure answer. Some research indicates that sunlight starts a chemical reaction in the plastic bottle that can result in carcinogens in the water.

How can you get pure water? I recommend a water purification system in your home or certified, chemical-free, spring-fed bottled water in glass containers.

An Essential Thing to Do

Drink eight cups of pure water each day.

#24

KNOW
WHY
YOU'RE
EATING

Long-term dietary changes require more than shifts in our menus. Our food preferences are a factor of culture and habit. Our enjoyment of food is so much a part of our lives that any permanent change must involve not only *what* we eat but also *why* we eat.

On countless occasions we allow our frame of mind, rather than our body, to determine our food choices. Comfort foods to satisfy our emotions, to soothe our anger, frustration, worry, boredom, or guilt, are most often the culprit. Relief from emotional distress is easily accomplished by eating. When this happens we have linked diet to emotional fulfillment. This is dangerous territory.

We need a heightened awareness of why we eat. Many patients who embark on the cancer recovery journey develop an attitude that changing their diet is something they *have* to do. Too bad. I suggest you try an outlook that reflects the fact that a change in diet is something you *get* to do!

Eating with awareness is easily accomplished with the help of these practices:

- Don't keep any high-fat snack foods around the house where they will be a serious temptation.
- Make a rule of not eating in front of the television, where you don't pay attention to what or how much you eat.
- Don't eat so quickly that you can't enjoy your food. It takes about twenty minutes for the brain to realize that the stomach is full. Slow down. Take a break mid-meal.
- Reward appropriate eating behavior, but don't use comfort foods as the reward. If you've had a good week or have reached a wellness goal, treat yourself to a movie, a concert, or a new outfit. Don't punish imperfection, just don't reward yourself. Try again next week.
- Make each meal a pleasant experience. Stop eating on the run or while standing at the kitchen counter. Take time to put out a place setting. Offer a short affirmation or prayer of gratitude for each meal. You'll then be nurturing yourself emotionally and spiritually, as well as physically.

An Essential Thing to Do

Distinguish between a food craving, which is a psychological need, and hunger, which is the body's need for nourishment. Check your urge to eat the next time you see a food advertisement. A craving diminishes when you take on another activity. Go for a walk. Call a friend. Read a book. Then evaluate. Were you feeling a craving or hunger? Honor your hunger, not your craving. Eat with awareness!

#25

DETERMINE YOUR NUTRITIONAL SUPPLEMENT PROGRAM

First and most important, if you have cancer, please immediately implement the following nutritional supplement program:

Each day consume 5,000 IU of vitamin D_3. Arrange for a monthly blood test. Adjust your vitamin D_3 consumption until you reach and maintain your 25(OH)D level at 55–60 ng/mL (nanograms per milliliter).

If you do not have cancer, consume 2,000 IU of vitamin D_3 each day as a preventative. Test your blood levels annually. Maintain a vitamin D level of 30–40 ng/mL.

Also, carefully study the guide entitled "The Vitamin D Promise" found in the back of this book.

Fact: Most cancer survivors believe in and use vitamin and mineral supplements.

Fiction: Vitamins are totally ineffective and should be avoided during cancer treatment.

The following food supplement guidelines, along with the whole foods, low fat/salt/sugar, fresh vegetable, and fresh fruit dietary strategy, form the basis for the Cancer Recovery Foundation's approach to nutrition. They are designed to guide and support people in ways to maximize strengthening the body and promoting an optimally functioning immune system.

I recommend that people take vitamin and mineral supplements. Exhaustive and credible research shows that the right levels of nutrients are both protective against developing many cancers as well as supportive of health and healing following a diagnosis.

Ideally we should receive all our nutrients from food. And vitamins cannot take the place of a healthy diet. But even with the best whole food diet, we may have trouble receiving all our required nutrients. Intensive farming practices have led to a demonstrated decline in the nutritional value of certain foods. The result is you may not receive all the nutrients you need in the right amounts all of the time.

In addition, increasing evidence of the negative impact of the wide range of chemicals we are exposed to in everyday life is significant. This calls for an even greater need for nutrients to help with detoxification and protection of the body's organs.

The following guidelines contain information about vitamins, minerals, and other nutritional supplements, along with recommended dosages, that are evidence-based and thought to be specifically supportive for people who have had a cancer diagnosis. Cancer Recovery Foundation developed this program to provide a full range of essential nutrients as well as obtain maximum absorption and bioavailability. For those people who wish to promote their general health and help prevent cancer, these guidelines are also helpful.

Research suggests that vitamins and minerals work best when combined in a way that they all work together, the action of one enhancing the action of others. A high-quality multivitamin and mineral supplement will contain a wide range of vitamins and minerals in levels that allow them to work effectively together. However, if the nutrient levels of your multivitamin are not as high as recommended, I suggest you supplement with individual doses of vitamins and minerals to reach Cancer Recovery Foundation's recommended dosage.

A SHORT OVERVIEW OF NUTRITIONAL SUPPLEMENTS AND CANCER

All essential nutrients are important for rebuilding and maintaining health. Research shows the following to be particularly beneficial to people with cancer.

Antioxidants

Antioxidants are the starting point. An antioxidant is a substance that prevents damage caused by excess free radicals in your body. Free radicals are highly reactive chemicals that can damage the DNA in our cells. DNA damage is known to be involved in the development of cancer.

The key antioxidant vitamins are C, E, and beta-carotene (a precursor of vitamin A). They work best in combination. They are especially beneficial in combating the effects of free radical damage to DNA. Selenium is an additional essential mineral that is an important part of antioxidant activity. And coenzyme Q10 is an antioxidant compound made naturally by the body and used by cells to produce controlled cell growth and maintenance. However, when the body's immune function is compromised, the body's natural ability to produce coQ10 is often impaired. These five vitamins and minerals form the basis of the Cancer Recovery Foundation's nutritional supplement program.

A common question is, "Why are the antioxidant doses the Cancer Recovery Foundation suggests higher than the government's Dietary Reference Intakes (DRIs)?" The DRI is often set at the level that prevents a deficiency disease, scurvy for example. But this does not necessarily mean that same level will be adequate for supporting maximum health, cancer prevention, or rebuilding the immune system of people with cancer. Cancer Recovery's guidelines meet standards above disease deficiency and therefore must be higher than the DRI.

Carotenoids

This is a class of natural pigments found principally in plants, algae, and certain bacteria. Carotenoids have antioxidant activity, and some, such as beta-carotene, are converted to vitamin A by the body. Lycopene is a particularly beneficial carotenoid for the prevention and natural treatment of cancer. Fresh organic tomatoes are a rich source of lycopene. In order to maximize absorption, tomatoes are best eaten lightly cooked, then pureed and topped with a splash of extra virgin olive oil.

Flavonoids

Like carotenoids, flavonoids are one of the groups of plant nutrients with powerful antioxidant characteristics as well as other cancer-fighting properties.

Omega-3 Fatty Acids

Three fatty acids—ALA (alpha-linolenic acid), DHA (docosahexaenoic acid), and EPA (eicosapentaenoic acid)—are essential to good health. For cancer patients, the fats are particularly important because they support immune function and hormone balance. The best source of the omega-3s is from oily fish, including wild salmon, tuna, mackerel, and sardines. For people unable or choosing not to eat fish, flaxseed oil can be a good source. However, flaxseed oil does not contain DHA or EPA. Some brands now add DHA from a plant source.

Probiotics

Probiotics are supplements of beneficial bacteria that promote gastrointestinal balance. One example is *Lactobacillus acidophilus*. Many cancer treatments are notorious for causing nausea and diarrhea. Most patients can find relief by rebalancing the intestinal tract with probiotics to maintain digestive health. A "detoxified" gastro-intestinal track also maximizes the removal of toxins from the body.

SUPPLEMENTS DURING TREATMENT

Taking supplements during cancer treatment is a subject of intense debate within the cancer community. Cancer Recovery Foundation carefully monitors international research on this subject, constantly updating our recommendations. Following consultation with your oncologist, we currently recommend:

- If you are on a chemotherapy regimen:
  - Continue your multivitamin but suspend your additional supplement program two days (forty-eight hours) prior to receiving treatment.
  - Recommence your additional supplement program three days (seventy-two hours) after receiving treatment.
  - If you are on a continuous infusion treatment protocol, continue your multivitamin but do not take additional supplements during your treatment.
- If you are on a radiation therapy or hormonal therapy regimen, continue to take your multivitamin and additional supplements throughout treatment.

OTHER NUTRITIONAL SUPPLEMENT ISSUES

Will you still need supplements following treatment? I am a believer. It is the Cancer Recovery Foundation's recommendation that all people with a personal history of cancer take supplements the remainder of their lives. Evidence is clear that proper nutrient levels translate to maximizing health and maintaining healing. In addition, we recommend that people taking supplements over their lifetimes have regular appointments with a nutritional therapist and check our Website, www.cancerrecovery .org, regularly for the most up-to-date nutritional guidelines.

I am frequently asked, "What brand name of supplements is best?" I do not have a good answer. I simply recommend you choose the highest-quality supplements available. The best supplements will contain fewer nonactive ingredients, such as preservatives and binding agents. Higher-quality supplements are also less likely to contain artificial sweeteners and coloring. While this level of supplement tends to be more expensive, I believe the incremental expense to be of value.

Some cancer patients have difficulty swallowing tablets. In fact, "pill burden" is experienced by approximately 25 percent of cancer patients. Simple techniques resolve nearly all these difficulties. Large tablets can be crushed. Capsules can be pierced (please note that lycopene products may stain the teeth). Many vitamins and minerals can be obtained in liquid and powder form. If your concern is complete absorption of the nutrients, choose sublingual products, which are designed to be absorbed under the tongue.

Finally, I would add that you need to keep up to date on nutritional supplement guidelines. Every three months Cancer Recovery Foundation monitors no less than sixteen different sources in twelve countries to review research findings on this important subject. We then review our recommendations and update them when evidence supports such changes.

CANCER RECOVERY FOUNDATION'S NUTRITIONAL SUPPLEMENTATION GUIDELINES

Supplement Recommendations and Dosages for People with Cancer

Note: Unless otherwise stated on the label, supplements are best taken with food in order to help maximize absorption.

Guidelines for all cancer patients during treatment and thereafter:

Nutrient	Details	Daily Dose	Comments
Multivitamin and mineral	Highest quality affordable	As directed on label	Minimal preservatives, binders, and sweeteners

Additional supplements for all cancer patients during treatment, and for two years following treatment, except as noted below:

Nutrient	Details	Daily Dose	Comments
Vitamin B	Part of multivitamin and mineral complex	50–100 mg	
Vitamin C with flavonoids	Nonacidic ascorbate forms or from foods	2,000 mg–2 g	Take amounts over 1 g in divided doses with meals.
Vitamin D_3	Be certain to take vitamin D_3 not vitamin D_2.	5,000 IU	Add to multivitamin to reach recommended dosage.
Vitamin E	Part of multivitamin and mineral complex	400 IU	Best taken with vitamin C and beta-carotene. *(Special note on vitamin E: If you have high blood pressure; are taking warfarin, aspirin, or any other anti-thrombotic drug; are on a chemotherapy regimen; or have a low platelet count, consult your doctor before taking more than 200 IU daily. This vitamin has a mild anticoagulant effect.)*
Beta-carotene	Part of multivitamin and mineral complex	25,000 IU	If you smoke or have smoked in the past ten years, do not take more than 2,000 IU daily.

Nutrient	Details	Daily Dose	Comments
Lycopene	Maximum of 7 mg when taken with beta-carotene	10–15 mg	Do not take carrot juice at the same time as lycopene.
Omega-3 fatty acid	Fish oils *Or . . .* Flaxseed oil with DHA	EPA + DHA 500 mg or more 1,000 mg	Whole fish oil. No cod oil, which may contain mercury. Vegan alternative for those allergic to fish.
Selenium	Part of multivitamin and mineral complex	200 mcg	
Zinc	Part of multivitamin and mineral complex	Women: 20 mg Men: 40 mg	
Coenzyme Q10	Protects heart during chemotherapy	100 mg	
Probiotics	For digestive disorder (nausea, diarrhea)	1 or 2 capsules, per label	Minimum 1 billion organisms. Keep refrigerated.
Milk thistle	For liver health during treatment	200 mg twice daily	

An Essential Thing to Do

Do your homework. Contact a professional nutritionist. Determine what specific experience he or she has in therapeutic nutritional supplementation for cancer. Compare the nutritionist's recommendations with Cancer Recovery Foundation's recommendations as well as your own research. Be skeptical of unsubstantiated claims. Then, make your own decisions regarding nutritional supplements.

Important Notice: These statements have not been evaluated by the Food and Drug Administration (FDA). Greg Anderson and Cancer Recovery Foundation make every effort to use up-to-date and reliable sources. However, we cannot accept liability for errors in the sources that we use. Also, we cannot guarantee to provide all the information that may be available concerning your individual health circumstances. All responsibility for interpretation of and action upon the information provided is yours. This information is offered on the understanding that if you intend to support your cancer treatment with complementary or alternative approaches, you will consult with your medical team to be certain they have a complete understanding of your choices.

#26

MAKE EXERCISE PART OF YOUR RECOVERY

Hundreds of cancer survivors helped me make an important discovery: Exercise directly correlates with health recovery. Nine out of ten people I interviewed talked about keeping physically active. Even people who were incapacitated or who needed a wheelchair emphasized their commitment to a regular exercise program.

Cancer survivors are markedly different, however, in their exercise goals. Very few set out to run a marathon or become Olympic athletes. Instead, the most common exercise goal among cancer survivors is to experience an increase in energy.

I chose walking as my exercise. At first I was so weak that even a couple of minutes of walking was too much. So I began with chair exercises, doing simple arm circles—the backstroke movement with my arms fully extended. I'd do ten sets forward and follow with ten sets in the reverse direction. Soon I felt that increase in energy—the deeper breathing, the increase in heart rate, and the better skin color.

It wasn't long before I began to feel stronger. It seemed exercise was working. So I added a few minutes of leg lifts. Soon I was strong enough to put walking back into my exercise routine. Initially, I walked for perhaps five minutes before feeling an increase in energy. But soon that time stretched to ten minutes. Over the months, the exercise periods became longer. I bought an exercise book and added some full-body stretching routines before the start of my walk, and I ended the exercise session with some light calisthenics. I began to feel the combination of physical and emotional regeneration working together to enhance my well-being. You can experience the same.

Today I believe I have found the right balance. Hardly a day passes that I do not walk for at least thirty minutes. I precede the walk with about three minutes of full-body stretches and conclude the session with five minutes of push-ups and sit-ups.

This did not happen overnight. I determined this to be my correct level over a period of two years. Several times I have experimented with exercise beyond the normal thirty-five- to forty-minute daily routine. I tried walking for an hour each day but found I was experiencing hip soreness. I tried weight lifting only to realize I didn't enjoy it.

Some people think more exercise is better. A gentleman recently wrote me to express his opinion that two hours of intense exercise each day is a requirement for cancer recovery. I don't recommend it. Between the threat of injury associated with extended exercise and the rigid, grinding routine that often results in burnout, I believe more harm than good can come from workouts that last two or three hours daily.

Instead, I recommend you find a type of exercise that you enjoy. Then practice that routine just until you feel an increase in energy. The benefits include increased flexibility, greater strength, more cardiovascular capacity, weight loss, and lower blood pressure. But the psychological benefits are even greater—joy, enthusiasm, and mental vitality. What a payoff!

Make exercise part of your cancer recovery program. No matter how long it has been since you have exercised, no matter how incapacitated or confined you are, there are exercises you can do. Exercise will help you get well again.

An Essential Thing to Do

Exercise just until you feel an increase in energy. This is your only exercise goal. Do the same tomorrow. Keep extending the duration as you build strength and stamina. No more excuses! Take charge. Your body will respond to this "get-well" signal.

#27

SLEEP
MORE

Fatigue. It's the most common complaint of cancer patients. "I'm always so tired. My radiation treatments drain me," noted Olivia during her recovery from breast cancer. "I just want to sleep all the time. But with all my responsibilities, who has time to sleep?"

Fatigue is part of nearly every cancer patient's experience. Unfortunately, many patients interpret fatigue as an indication of their fast-approaching demise. Not so!

During and just after treatment, you are a different person physically. Just consider what is happening to you. With surgery, a major wound has been inflicted on your body. Chemotherapy puts chemicals into your system that alter your unique biochemical makeup. Radiation causes genetic and cellular changes in your body. Repairs demand rest. No wonder cancer patients are tired.

"For three months I cut back to half days at work," said Ted Chadwick after his bout with bladder cancer. "I took an afternoon nap for a year following my treatment." shared Alicia, who recovered from ovarian cancer. "I still take afternoon naps," said Bert

Byer, celebrating his six-year anniversary of a lung cancer diagnosis.

The fact is, survivors rest. I previously mentioned ginseng as an assist to overcome fatigue. However, no supplement or medication is a replacement for sleep. It is a major mistake to carry on at the same frantic pace to which you were accustomed when you were supposedly healthy. Feeling tired is normal for anyone with any illness. During treatment you may feel tired for weeks until your body gets the opportunity to adjust and recover. So allow yourself rest.

Provided you are getting adequate food and moderate exercise, fatigue is nothing to consume you with worry. It is not a sure sign of your demise. Take that morning nap. Add an afternoon nap if you require it. Or a short rest before dinner may be just what is needed. Eight or more hours of sleep each night is an absolute essential.

An Essential Thing to Do

Give yourself permission to get more sleep. Block out rest times on your wellness schedule. Allow your body the rest it needs to repair and heal.

#28

FIND
POSITIVE
SUPPORT

Fact: Cancer patients who regularly participate in support group meetings live longer than those who do not.

Ongoing research at Stanford University confirmed what cancer survivors have known for decades. In a study of patients with advanced breast cancer, those who attended a weekly two-hour support group session had a life expectancy twice that of the non-attenders. Further research at UCLA and King's College in London confirms the value of attending support groups. The message is clear: we truly need one another for survival.

Distinguish between the two major types of support groups: clinical and psychosocial. The clinical groups communicate basic knowledge on a wide variety of oncology issues. Subjects might include types of cancer treatments, common side effects, physical therapy following breast surgery, or how to live with an ostomy. The idea behind this type of support group is simply to inform.

More critical to survival are the psychosocial support groups. These are the supportive/expressive therapeutic programs that focus on the emotional, psychological, and spiritual aspects of cancer. Look for groups that take a stance of hope without denying the reality of the illness. At meetings you should expect to express your own fears and frustrations freely and allow others in the group to do the same. You'll learn from the responses of the group members who have overcome cancer, and you'll contribute to those who are just beginning the cancer recovery journey.

Does a support group make a difference? Women with breast cancer are the largest group of female survivors of cancer. Not surprisingly, women with breast cancer are also the most frequent attendees at cancer support groups. In a landmark study, letters of invitation were mailed to 1,336 breast cancer survivors who had participated in an earlier survey and support group activities. They were now between five and ten years after their initial diagnosis.

The 914 respondents were then sent a survey booklet that assessed a broad range of quality of life and survivorship concerns. A total of 817 women completed the follow-up survey. The findings include:

- Physical well-being and emotional well-being were excellent; the minimal changes between the baseline and follow-up assessments reflected expected age-related changes.
- Energy level and social functioning were unchanged.
- Hot flashes, night sweats, vaginal discharge, and breast sensitivity were decreased.
- Symptoms of vaginal dryness and urinary incontinence were increased.
- Sexual activity with a partner declined significantly.
- Survivors with no past systemic adjuvant therapy had a better quality of life than those who had received chemotherapy, tamoxifen, or both together.

At the Stanford School of Medicine, the effects of weekly supportive group meetings for women with breast cancer were systematically evaluated in a one-year, randomized, prospective outcome study.

This was talk therapy. The groups focused on the problems of illness, including improving relationships with family and friends and living as fully as possible in the face of cancer. The investigators hypothesized that this support group intervention would lead to improved mood, coping strategies, and self-esteem among those in the treatment group.

Eighty-six patients were tested at four-month intervals. The treatment groups had significantly lower mood-disturbance scores on the Profile of Mood States scale, had fewer coping problems, and were less phobic than the control group.

These studies provide objective evidence that support group participation results in psychological benefits and improved quality of life.

One warning: A potential problem with any type of support group is that instead of encouraging personal growth, many groups quickly turn into a "pity party." While there is significant value in allowing people to talk out their problems, the discerning group needs a leader to judge when the talking is therapeutic and when it is rehearsing, and reinforcing, a problem. The "cybersolace" provided in online chat groups is no exception.

When a group of us started Cancer Conquerors support groups, committing to support one another in our wellness quests, we made a pact early on. Each meeting would include a lesson—somebody leading a discussion on a recovery principle—and a time for open discussion and support. The emphasis was to be on the application of lessons that would help contribute to our own healing. It was the smartest move we ever made. We have experienced very few pity parties.

An Essential Thing to Do

Contact Cancer Recovery Foundation at www.cancerrecovery.org. A full schedule of our unique Cancer Conqueror Telesupport groups exists. Experience several. Then judge for yourself.

If you don't find what you are looking for, perhaps you need to consider starting a group in your home. Thousands of patients have done so, benefiting themselves and others in their community. Contact Cancer Recovery Foundation of America for start-up information.

THE FIFTH STEP:
HEAL
WITH THE
MIND

Do personal beliefs, positive attitudes, and hopeful expectations make a contribution to cancer recovery? A great deal of credible scientific evidence says "Yes." In fact, the contribution may be greater than science has the ability to measure.

Fighting cancer is much, much more than simply excising a tumor, exposing a malignancy to radiation, or administering chemotherapy through an intravenous drip.

Think bigger. Imagine harnessing all your resources, including the mind/body connection. The basics are actually quite simple. Let's continue our work.

#29

STUDY
THESE
RESOURCES

Anderson, Greg. *The Cancer Conqueror*. Dallas: Word, 1988. And *Cancer and the Lord's Prayer*. Des Moines: Meredith Books, 2006. Two of my messages of hope and encouragement found through the body-mind-spirit connection.

Benson, Herbert, and Miriam Klipper. *The Relaxation Response*. New York: Quill, 2001. The definitive source for relaxation and meditation concepts and techniques.

Borysenko, Joan. *Minding the Body, Mending the Mind*. New York: Da Capo Lifelong, 2007. How to manage stressful thoughts and uncertainty.

Lerner, Michael. *Choices in Healing: Integrating the Best of Conventional and Complementary Approaches to Cancer*. Cambridge, MA: MIT Press, 1994. The intellectual's guide to alternative treatments.

LeShan, Lawrence. *Cancer as a Turning Point*. New York: Plume, 1994. The emotional aspects of cancer. Helpful exercises involving reflection, discussion, and writing to help come to terms with fears.

Siegel, Bernie. *Love, Medicine & Miracles*. New York: HarperPerennial, 1990. Stories about self-healing from a former surgeon's observations of cancer patients.

Simonton, O. Carl, Stephanie Matthews-Simonton and James Creighton. *Getting Well Again*. Los Angeles: J. P. Tarcher, 1978. Guides cancer patients to participate in recovery through imagery and therapy.

An Essential Thing to Do

Visit your bookseller or library. Become immersed in mobilizing your mind for healing.

#30

ANALYZE YOUR BELIEFS

Millions of cancer survivors radically change their beliefs about cancer and about life. Many consider this to be the most fundamental aspect of healing with the mind. I urge you to understand that this idea has a central place in your own recovery efforts.

There are three widely held cultural beliefs that work against overcoming cancer:

1. A diagnosis of cancer means my certain death.
2. The treatment of cancer is drastic, is of questionable effectiveness, and involves many side effects.
3. This diagnosis "just happened" to me, and therefore, there is little I can do to influence it.

All of the above beliefs are untrue! The truth about these statements is:

1. Cancer, no matter how advanced, may or may not mean death.

2. A wide range of treatments do exist and have the potential to be effective. The difficulties in recovery are far outweighed by the benefits.
3. Most illnesses do not "just happen." Our ability to influence health is significant.

These truths can work for you in your recovery. Your response to a problem is more powerful than the problem itself. There is much you can do.

Beliefs have a powerful effect over physical realities. Our beliefs affect the way we perceive illness and literally control our response to it. Beliefs are the determinant of emotions that have a direct link to physical health. In short, our beliefs about ourselves, our disease, our treatment, and our role in healing are inextricably linked with outcomes.

Consciously or unconsciously, our beliefs are creating our reality. It's true both positively and negatively. After interviewing over 16,000 cancer survivors, I know of no survivors who believed that they could not get well. I also have observed that survivors come to understand that beliefs are just thoughts. Thoughts can be changed. If we can bring ourselves to see the central role of beliefs, we can then create self-fulfilling prophecies based on non-limiting beliefs.

Do beliefs affect recovery? Consider this. Beliefs and expectations constantly contribute to actual experiences in all areas of life, including the experience of cancer. If we believe a rainy day means gloom, gloom is what we experience.

I realize it's a long way from rainy days to cancer recovery. But this much is clear: beliefs can be chosen. The sad fact is we seldom consciously choose them. Perhaps beliefs have simply been accepted by us for many years, like the conventional wisdom surrounding cancer. Perhaps we had beliefs imposed from parents, coworkers, or friends. We may have picked up other people's beliefs and made them our own. They may or may not be true or helpful. But these beliefs have significant power.

Awareness of our fundamental beliefs is often the first, and certainly one of the most dramatic ways to improve our circumstances. If you are harboring the belief that cancer means death, challenge it! The fact is, there are long-term survivors of every type of cancer, including many patients who have been told by doctors that there was no hope.

An Essential Thing to Do

Carefully analyze your beliefs. In your Wellness and Recovery Journal, complete the following sentences with the first thoughts/feelings that come to mind:

1. One belief I hold about my cancer diagnosis is_____

_____

2. One belief I hold about my cancer treatment is_____

_____

3. One belief I hold about my role in survival is_____

_____

Analyze how your beliefs align with the truths. Talk to others who have successfully traveled the cancer journey. Discover what they believe. Vow to change your self-limiting beliefs today.

#31

"REFRAME"
YOUR CANCER

If you're like most cancer patients, you look upon your illness as the most overwhelming threat to your life you've ever encountered. "I thought of cancer as a powerful evil and deadly force inflicting great injury on me," said Raymond Valrico, a retired restaurant owner who was battling cancer of the larynx. "It was the ultimate threat."

Raymond's words describe his mental outlook. *Cancer . . . a powerful evil and deadly force . . . inflicting great injury . . . the ultimate threat.* It took weeks of counseling, but Raymond came to view his cancer not as a threat but as a *challenge.* Cancer became something that stimulated him to introspection, to review his life. Raymond ultimately made changes in his exercise routine, diet, vocation, and spiritual life. Cancer became Raymond's wake-up call.

Raymond's experience is a perfect example of what it means to reframe the illness. Reframing is the process of finding alternative ways, more positive means, of viewing and responding to any circumstance.

Jose Padilla's diagnosis of prostate cancer was the most frightening and unwelcome event in his fifty-eight years. Even though tests confirmed that the cancer had been discovered early and the prognosis was quite optimistic, his chronic panic-driven thought process focused on his imminent demise. "I don't just have cancer, I was cancer," said Jose.

Frank Cummins also had prostate cancer, but his was significantly more advanced than Jose's. Frank had bone involvement. Unlike Jose, Frank made the critical distinction that he had cancer, the cancer did not have him. "I realized that my mind and spirit had cancer only if I allowed it." Frank's outlook reframed the cancer.

Frank's response demonstrates the significant power we possess. The point of control is not the circumstance of illness; it is our response to the illness. Our response can make all the difference. When we reframe cancer, we respond differently and more proactively. We acknowledge and nourish our inner strength, even in the face of doubt and fear. The threat subsides. We take on the challenge.

Fortunately, both stories have happy endings. Jose was able to embrace many of Frank's more positive beliefs. Today both men are doing well.

An Essential Thing to Do

Examine your core beliefs. Then follow this reframing process:

1. What belief about cancer do I want to change?_____

_____

2. What does holding this belief currently gain me?_____

_____

3. How might I come to view cancer as an inspiring challenge rather than a threat?_____

_____

Remember, challenges inspire you to action. Respond to the challenge of cancer.

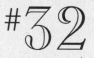

Evaluate
Your
Self-Talk

From the moment we awaken in the morning until we drift off to sleep at night, we experience a constant stream of mental chatter. When we have cancer, our "self-talk" is nearly all negative, filled with fears. It makes for a frightening life experience.

Marion Bricker called Cancer Recovery Foundation in a state of panic, her mind reeling out of control. After the first couple of minutes, I began to jot down the opening phrases of her sentences. They gave a clear picture of her state of mind:

"The cancer is spreading . . ." "I think my insurance is going to be canceled . . ." "How am I going to pay for this?" "It's all such a burden . . ." "I'm afraid of chemotherapy . . ." "My husband can't deal with this . . ." "I feel so frightened . . ." "Why did this happen to me?" "Where is God when you need him?" "There's nothing I can do."

Yes, there is something Marion can do! And you can, too. Believe it or not, we absolutely do choose our every thought. We may think the same fear-filled thought over and over, out of habit, but we are still responsible for that original choice. Analyze the thoughts you have been holding about cancer. That self-talk is the ancestor of your current experience of illness.

Lou Lafferty is a woman who has every excuse needed to lead a life of despair. Childhood abuse, a turbulent early marriage, children in trouble, a toxic divorce, a child who ran away, a second husband who died in a work accident, a serious auto accident after which she was disabled for eight months, and then lymphoma. "My mind," explained Lou, "was always filled with thoughts of life being unfair and difficult, a battle."

Then Lou discovered this great truth: self-talk can change every life experience.

Lou made massive changes. First, she came to the profound realization that her troubles were all in her past, over and done. What happened in the past did not automatically predict what would happen in the future. Of primary importance, Lou came to realize that the thoughts and words she chose right here and now were the ones creating her future. Her self-talk set in place her experience, either good or bad.

That was thirteen years ago. Today Lou is cancer-free, a happy, healthy, and whole person.

An Essential Thing to Do

Complete this awareness-builder. Write down a positive empowering message you can give yourself in the following circumstances.

Circumstance: You're frustrated with the doctor for his arrogance, his impatience with your questions, and the limited amount of time he spends with you.

*Positive self-talk:*_____

_____

Circumstance: It's 3:00 AM and you're wide awake, consumed with thoughts and fears of suffering and self-pity.

*Positive self-talk:*_____

_____

Circumstance: Your energy level is at an all-time low. You are tired and discouraged, questioning if you can take any more.

*Positive self-talk:*_____

_____

Notice what you are thinking at this moment. Is your self-talk negative or positive? Do you wish for your future to be an extension of these thoughts?

#33

Choose a Daily Affirmation

Affirmations are positive statements of intent and belief. They take the place of the negative mental chatter that may be gripping you. Affirmations serve to "make firm" the positive things about you and your circumstances. They are consciously chosen self-talk.

Your words are constantly doing one of two things: building you up or tearing you down, healing or destroying. So affirm positively. You are not so much changing the situation as you are changing your thinking about the situation. Changing your thinking about the disease of cancer may be at the heart of experiencing wellness.

Self-talk is the constant conversation of our minds. We process everything, our internal dialogue always interpreting events and creating meaning. Positive affirmations can guide and direct this inner conversation and, in the process, change our response. Affirmations are simply short statements that express the desired outcome. When combined with an acceptance that the old belief is changeable, and the genuine desire to change, we begin to create a new reality.

Affirmations are most powerful when expressed in the present tense. The phrase "I am grateful for life today" is much preferred over a future-tense alternative like, "I will show gratitude for my life."

Positive affirmations were first brought to notice in the Western medical world by Emile Coue, a nineteenth-century French pharmacist who noticed that several of his patients dramatically improved when they focused on positive health outcomes rather than the negative fears and images of illness. Coue's famous affirmation, which he encouraged his patients to use, lives on today: *Every day, in every way, I am getting better and better.*

However, affirmations can be exceedingly difficult to believe. It's one of the central reasons that positive thinking is sometimes limited in its effect. An exclusive focus on the positive can result in a sense of unreality. For example, if you have a strong inner belief that you are a bad person and disease is your rightful punishment, telling yourself that you are going to get well is probably not going to work. Predictably, it will be necessary to first recognize the underlying beliefs and challenge the negative ones before the positive ones can be effective.

Affirmation has been dismissed by some people in the medical community as brainwashing. In a way, it is. For years we may have been brainwashing ourselves with limiting beliefs such as, "I am a bad person." When you substitute an opposite and non-limiting belief such as, "I am a child of God, worthy of all God's best," you are deliberately washing your brain with what may seem to be, at first, an artificial construct.

This artificiality is often a problem at first. For example, the affirmation "I am cancer-free" sounds pretty ridiculous when you've just been given the negative results of a CT scan. But the key is to initially pretend, to play with the new belief as if it were true. Our minds cannot yet accept a belief that contradicts the old limits. But it can accept a kind of imagery game in which we play with the new belief as if it were reality. And it is through the play and practice that the new belief gradually becomes believable.

Then we must act. Putting the new desired belief into action confirms and strengthens it. In a spiritual sense, this is acting on faith. You begin to believe that your new belief can be reality and so you act as if it is. At first you do this in very small ways, setting easily attainable goals.

I changed my health with one very powerful affirmation. Right in the middle of the cancer battle, starting at the point where I was down to 112 pounds, confined to bed, and on morphine to control the pain, I began to affirm:

"I am cancer-free, a picture of health. Thank you, God."

I coupled this spoken affirmation with a mental picture of pink healthy cells, a smile on my face, an image of being vital and alive, and my outstretched hands held over my head giving thanks to God. If you came to our home today, you would see a photo of me on a beach, hands lifted overhead, greeting a new day and affirming a new and healthy life.

I would repeat this affirmation countless times—300, 400, even 500 times a day. I'd whisper it. I say it in a normal tone of voice. I'd shout it out loud—at least when no one was at home.

I credit this work of speaking health and healing into my life as the point of power that turned the tide in my cancer journey. Make affirmations work for you. Change your mind and you'll change your health. Whatever we affirm tends to become manifest in our lives. Why not affirm the very best, not out of blindness to illness but out of the well-founded hope of creating your own positive self-fulfilling prophecies of wellness.

Here's how to challenge beliefs and make affirmations work for you:

1. Understand and accept that the old belief is not reality.
2. Nurture a genuine desire to change.
3. Substitute the old belief with the new affirmation.
4. Combine the positive affirmation with positive action.

An Essential Thing to Do

Study the following examples. Implement them in your own healing program.

#1 Limiting Belief
CANCER MEANS DEATH. *Similar beliefs:* Cancer cells are powerful. I am always ill. My body is weak. My resistance is low. I might struggle but the cancer will eventually get me.
Non-limiting Affirmation
CANCER IS A MESSAGE TO CHANGE. *Similar affirmations:* Cancer cells are weak and confused. I have a healthy body. I am building my immune function. My body has its own inner healing wisdom.

#2 Limiting Belief
CANCER TREATMENTS ARE TOXIC AND INEFFECTIVE. *Similar beliefs:* I hate my treatments. I always get sick after treatment. I am always so tired after radiation.
Non-limiting Affirmation
I CHOOSE TREATMENTS THAT HAVE MY "EXCITED" BELIEF. *Similar affirmations:* I believe in my minimally invasive treatment choices. My treatment side effects are readily managed. I am filled with healing energy.

#3 Limiting Belief
THERE IS NOTHING I CAN DO. *Similar beliefs:* I am a victim of cancer. I have no control over what happens to me. I can't help what I think. I can't help what I feel. I have no choice.
Non-limiting Affirmation
I AM IN CHARGE OF MY CANCER. *Similar affirmations:* There is a great deal that I can do. I am in charge of my own life. I have many choices. I have great creative resources.

#4 Limiting Belief
I AM SO AFRAID. *Similar beliefs:* I am helpless. I am trapped. I fear surgery . . . chemotherapy . . . radiation.
Non-limiting Affirmation
I AM FILLED WITH HOPE. *Similar affirmations:* I am confident. God's spirit of love is within me. I have positive choices.

#5 Limiting Belief
I DON'T HAVE ANY ENERGY. *Similar beliefs:* It's too hard for me. I am lazy.
Non-limiting Affirmation
I AM ACTIVE. *Similar affirmations:* I have positive energy. Joy and pleasure help me heal.

#6 Limiting Belief
IT'S GOING TO TURN OUT BADLY. *Similar beliefs:* I'm unhappy. There's no hope. I don't deserve healing.
Non-limiting Affirmation
THIS IS GOING TO TURN OUT PERFECTLY. *Similar affirmations:* I am happy. Life is good. I am worthy of healing. I accept myself as I am now.

#7 Limiting Belief
I AM A WEAK PERSON. *Similar beliefs:* I am emotionally . . . intellectually . . . physically . . . spiritually weak. I am not capable of self-healing.
Non-limiting Affirmation
I AM STRONG. *Similar affirmations:* I am filled with "heart." I am filled with self-respect. I have a fighting spirit.

#8 Limiting Belief
I'M NOT GOOD ENOUGH IN GOD'S EYES. *Similar beliefs:* I'm not worthy. I'm not acceptable to God. I am always wrong . . . guilty . . . inferior . . . a failure. God is out to "get" me.
Non-limiting Affirmation
GOD DEEPLY LOVES ME. *Similar affirmations:* I am a good person. God created me. I am a child of God. I accept myself as I am. I respect myself.

#9 Limiting Belief
MY DOCTORS DON'T CARE ABOUT ME. *Similar beliefs:* People don't really care. Healthcare professionals are only out for

what they can get. My doctor rejects me. My doctor cares only about his/her fee.

Non-limiting Affirmation
PEOPLE LIKE AND CARE FOR ME. *Similar affirmations:* My doctor did what he/she did with the best possible motives. He/She really does care for me. I care for myself.

#10 Limiting Belief
THINGS WILL NEVER GET BETTER. *Similar beliefs:* Things never change. Things are getting worse. I can never change. People in my life can never change. I'll never have the healing I want.

Non-limiting Affirmation
EVERY DAY, IN EVERY WAY, I AM GETTING BETTER AND BETTER. *Similar affirmations:* Everything is changing for the better. My healing goes well. I feel good about myself. God is for me. Life is good. This day is good. I am worthy of all God's blessings.

#34

MANAGE
YOUR
TOXIC
STRESS

Toxic stress is emotional overload. It is not the circumstances we are experiencing nor is it simply our negative emotions. Toxic stress is the *perception* of overload, the overflow of emotions, sometimes expressed but many times suppressed. This perception is experienced in our minds independent of the circumstances. Importantly, this perception is under our complete control.

Toxic stress only adds to the physical and mental anguish cancer brings. Stress works at cross-purposes to wellness, putting the mind in a state of confusion, blurring the focused peacefulness needed for healing.

There is something you can do about this perception. It's called the "relaxation response." First named and described by Herbert Benson, M.D., a cardiologist and associate professor of medicine at Harvard Medical School, the relaxation response is a simple, effective, self-healing meditation technique for reducing the detrimental effects of all kinds of stress that we live with every day, particularly the stress associated with a life-threatening illness.

Dr. Benson found that the relaxation response is even more

effective when one chooses a focus word or phrase that is closely tied to one's spiritual beliefs. The idea is to pick a word or short passage that has meaning for you: a Christian might use *The Lord is my Shepherd* from the Twenty-third Psalm; a Jewish person might choose *shalom;* a nonreligious phrase might be used, such as the word *peace.*

Pick a phrase with significant personal meaning. Dr. Benson calls this the "faith factor" and explains that it can greatly contribute to helping our minds manage stress more effectively.

The quest for daily self-renewal starts with a decision to handle our problems with a sense of equanimity. Eliciting the relaxation response, especially when coupled with the faith factor, results in our minds working for, rather than against, our wellness.

An Essential Thing to Do

Triggering the relaxation response is simple. Try these steps:

1. Find a quiet place, free from distractions, and sit in a comfortable position.
2. Pick a focus word or short phrase that is deeply rooted in your spiritual beliefs.
3. Close your eyes and relax your muscles, from toe to head, particularly relaxing the shoulder and neck area where most tension is carried.
4. Breathe slowly and naturally. Repeat your focus word silently as you exhale.
5. Assume a passive attitude. When a distracting thought comes to mind, simply dismiss it and return to your focus word.
6. Practice this response for ten to twenty minutes twice a day.

In your Wellness and Recovery Journal, check your daily schedule. Do you have time blocked, twice a day, for stress management? Schedule it. Honor these appointments.

#35

VISUALIZE
HEALTH AND
HEALING

An extension of the relaxation process is visualization, also known as mental imagery. This is a valuable tool for helping you reinforce belief in a desired outcome. It is an extension of the relaxation exercises in that it is typically added at or near the end of the meditation period.

The essence of visualization is to 1) create mental pictures of your immune system and of your treatment effectively fighting the cancer. You then 2) visualize the cancer disappearing and your body returning to health. Visualization is that simple, there's no need to make it any more complicated. I urge you to try it.

Consider some of these guidelines: Picture the cancer in symbolic images. For those who require a realistic image, you may want to consult an anatomy text to find pictures of actual cancer cells. Most patients, however, use symbols. I've had people describe their cancer as sand, a lump of clay, and even ice cubes. I saw mine as jelly. The most important criterion for picturing the disease is to think of the cancer as weak and confused. Don't give it power. Your imagery need not be anatomically correct unless you hold a belief that images of correct anatomy are required. What is important is the meaning you give the cancer's imagined symbol; visualize the cancer as weak.

Imagine your treatment as strong and powerful, damaging only the weak cancer cells. Imagine your healthy cells remaining intact. Picture your immune system fighting the cancer. Imagine the weak and damaged cancer cells being naturally flushed out of your body. Picture the cancer shrinking until it is gone. If you are experiencing pain, picture your white blood cells flowing to that area and soothing the pain. Whatever the problem, give your body the command to heal itself, visualizing the process in a way that makes sense to you. End the imagery by seeing yourself well, free of disease, and filled with energy.

How has this benefited you? Most people's fears tend to decrease as the imagery process gives them a greater sense of control. Ongoing research leads us to believe the imagery process has an influence on the body, actually triggering a hormonal and biochemical response to a renewed sense of hope. The resulting changes to the body's chemistry influence immune function, thus assisting the body in maximizing its opportunity to heal.

Science is proving the efficacy of visualization. Studies have shown that by practicing guided imagery a person is able to:

- temporarily increase numbers of immune system cells
- help reduce feelings of depression
- increase feelings of well-being

In studies of breast cancer patients, guided imagery has been shown to boost immunoglobulin A, an immune system precursor. In these same patients, visualization was also reported to relieve anxiety, depression, and moodiness.

In a study conducted at Oregon Health and Science University published in 2002, twenty-five women with stages I and II breast cancer were led through guided imagery sessions. During the sessions, the women were encouraged to imagine certain kinds of protective immune system cells—called natural killer cells—

finding, destroying, and removing cancer cells. The initial session was taped. The women used the tapes to practice at home three times a week for eight weeks.

Researchers measured the women's immune function and emotional state immediately before the program began, immediately after the eight-week sessions and then three months after the program ended. After combining these results, researchers found that the women had less depression and higher natural killer cell counts. However, while the women had more natural killer cells, the activity of those cells was not very different than it had been originally.

In a British study, ninety-six women with breast cancer were split into two groups. Both groups received traditional cancer care including six cycles of chemotherapy. But one group also received relaxation training and guided imagery. The women in the guided imagery group experienced better quality of life and easier expression of emotions than the group receiving only the traditional care.

In a Korean study published in 2005, thirty breast cancer patients were given progressive relaxation training and taught to use guided imagery during their six months of chemotherapy. Another thirty patients were treated with chemotherapy alone. The group practicing progressive relaxation and guided imagery experienced less nausea and vomiting, and they were less anxious, depressed, and irritable than the group receiving chemotherapy alone. Six months after treatment ended the progressive relaxation and guided imagery group was still experiencing a better quality of life than the group that did not receive training.

A recent review of forty-six studies found guided imagery to be helpful in managing stress, anxiety, and depression and in lowering blood pressure, reducing pain, and reducing some side effects of chemotherapy. Another review noted that guided imagery was helpful for anxiety as well as anticipatory nausea and vomiting from chemotherapy. Anticipatory or conditioned nausea and vomiting is when patients experience these problems before the next dose is given.

But not all studies have been positive on visualization's effects. A 2006 review of clinical trials of imagery found that only three studies showed improvement in anxiety and comfort during chemotherapy. Two other studies showed no difference between those who used imagery and those who used other measures.

Even with these mixed results, guided imagery is considered the single most useful psychological tool to reduce the side effects of chemotherapy.

Visualization is controversial. More than a few healthcare professionals consider it to be a form of self-deception. "After all," they reason, "I can show you that the tumor has been growing."

I encourage you to consider this response. In your own mind, separate what is happening from what you wish the outcome to be. It is possible, and beneficial, to picture the cancer shrinking even though it may, at this moment, be growing. This is not self-deception. It is self-direction, and it is necessary to begin the pursuit of any life goal. At first, reality will lag behind the vision you have of the desired outcome. But that vision will tend to pull you in the direction you need to go.

How can you make this technique work for you? After evoking the relaxation response, try this:

1. Picture your cancer cells as weak and confused.
2. Create a mental image of your treatment and your immune system overcoming the cancer.
3. Imagine your body's natural processes eliminating the disease from your system.
4. Envision the cancer shrinking until it disappears.
5. Imagine yourself well, filled with vitality for living.

An Essential Thing to Do

Evoke the relaxation response. End it with a visualization exercise. Do so at least twice daily.

Maximize
Mind, Body,
and Treatment

Conventional wisdom holds that cancer treatments are ineffective and have drastic side effects. Don't believe it. Conventional wisdom needs to be challenged.

Here's the truth: cancer treatments are becoming more effective every day. Treatments are also becoming more disease-targeted, affecting fewer healthy cells. I think primarily of proton beam radiation therapy. Plus, several new drugs hold promise for lessening the severity of many of the negative side effects.

Vitally important is the mind's role in combating side effects. In an experiment of a new chemotherapy, part of the group was given saline solution, sterile saltwater, as a placebo. Fully 30 percent of this group lost their hair! It is common for patients to experience nausea, not during or after treatment, but on their way to treatment; this is known as anticipatory nausea. Add to this the legions of examples in which the same treatment results in radically different side effects for different patients, and what do you get? Even allowing for physiological differences, the mind is at work; our beliefs are turned into biological realities.

You and I may perceive our cancer treatments entirely differently. During one of our Cancer Recovery Workshops, I asked Carol, a nursing-home administrator, to draw a picture illustrating her body, her breast cancer, and her treatment.

A few minutes later, she returned with a drawing of a huge devil injecting a charred and smoldering breast with a large syringe of poison. At that same seminar, Rhoda told us that she initially refused both chemotherapy and radiation because she saw them as highly toxic, more threatening than cancer itself. When I asked Rhoda to draw a similar picture, both of her chemotherapy and her radiation therapy, she returned with drawings of chemotherapy as acid eating through a tabletop and radiation therapy as a beam of light that was blinding her vision.

Let's conduct a self-administered evaluation. I ask you to stop your work for a moment, lay down this book, and find a piece of paper and a pencil. Now take a moment to illustrate:

1. Your body
2. The cancer
3. Your treatment

If you have not done so, please do so now.

Now, carefully observe what you have drawn. This is how you are currently representing your cancer experience. And if you believe mind affects body, the implications of these images are very significant. There is more detailed information on this important subject in the Guide entitled "Illness Representations" located in the back of this book.

Negative perceptions of treatment stand in the way of the body's ability to respond favorably. Whenever a patient sees treatment as a friend, a more positive perception starts to work favorably with the treatment. The best way to make treatment a friend is to make certain you "own" the treatment program, knowing that this is what you consider to be the very best course of action at this time.

Your mind is the key. You can program yourself for the most

positive outcome possible by using a type of visualization that athletes have successfully employed in training. After evoking the relaxation response, picture yourself sitting in a chair or lying on a table having your treatment administered. In your mind's eye, see the cancer shrinking. Feel your strength returning. At the end of your imaginary treatment, you feel good and ready to enjoy the gifts of renewed health and greater well-being.

If you do this frequently, especially during your course of treatment, evidence suggests your body will respond to the actual treatment with maximum capacity and minimal side effects. Like an Olympic athlete, you will be living the event in your mind first. Your mind helps the body get the message as to how it is expected to respond in the actual situation.

An Essential Thing to Do

View your treatment as a friend. Take time, make time, to "imagine" your treatment dramatically helping you. Envision yourself as well, free of any treatment side effects, and returning to radiant health.

The steps in this section are basic and fundamental mind/body principles. There's much more to healing with the mind. You may want to continue your training with more reading, attending seminars and workshops, and perhaps personalized instruction. Start with the source list in section 29. Or contact the Cancer Recovery Foundation at www.cancerrecovery.org.

THE SIXTH STEP: EMBRACE YOUR NEW LIFE

It is perhaps difficult to imagine any benefit coming from the experience of cancer. With the frightening diagnosis, the myriad of treatment decisions, and the need to manage all the negative side effects, how could cancer ever be a force for good?

Hundreds of thousands of survivors tell of the real and lasting changes that come directly from their cancer journey. A whole new and better chapter of life has opened before them. I wish this for you, too.

#37

UNDERSTAND
THE
MESSAGE
OF ILLNESS

When you "reframed" cancer, you began to see illness as more of a challenge than a threat. Now it is time to take this exercise one step further.

The challenge in illness can be found in its message to change. In a real sense, the challenge and message of cancer is a call, an opportunity, for personal growth. In this reframe of cancer lies the seed of true healing and lasting well-being.

Could cancer be a message signaling you to make changes in your life? We've already suggested several changes on the physical level—diet, exercise, and lifestyle issues. Might there be more?

Many survivors view cancer as a call for personal transformation. The changes go beyond physical health habits to changes in attitude and self-image. The wise patient uses the experience of cancer as a turning point, a time to replace ineffective and limited ways of coping by substituting healthier, more effective methods of nurturing relationships, developing vocations, and pursuing spiritual growth.

However, as soon as I suggest this position, people cry, "On some level, you're suggesting I subconsciously gave myself cancer!" Not so! We may have participated, but we did not purposely set out to give ourselves a serious illness. Don't read blame, self-sabotage, or guilt into the message of illness. Instead, realize the changes are potential points of power. Understand that if we have participated in our illness, even subconsciously, then we can participate in our wellness.

Many patients who sincerely explore the message of illness often discover a link between their physical, emotional, and even spiritual states of well-being and the onset of their illness. More important, a large number of the survivors whom I have interviewed can trace the beginning of their healing to their decision to change these beliefs and behaviors. They were able to examine the hidden message in illness and choose a response that changed their lives.

I believe that all of us have a personal responsibility to respond to cancer in this manner. Such a response is in your personal power. Start by asking yourself the following questions:

- *What high-stress events or changes happened in the year or two prior to diagnosis?* Become keenly aware of uncontrollable misfortunes. Death of a spouse or child, loss of a job, and financial setbacks are obvious candidates. Also include internal stresses, such as disappointments, major life adjustments, and ongoing conflict in important personal relationships. Most survivors can identify one or more major stresses in their lives prior to the onset of cancer.

- *What was my emotional response to these circumstances?* Did you process your grief over the loss, express your emotions, and finally adopt a hopeful stance, or did you sink into a chronic depressed state? This is a measure of your participation. Don't read blame here. Participation simply refers to how you responded to the circumstances that may have triggered the stress. Might you have put others' needs before your own? Did you give yourself permission to mourn the loss or did you determine you were going to be invincible and show no emotions? Did you permit yourself to seek the support of others during these stresses? How effective was your emotional self-care? Many survivors gain significant insight from a close examination of these questions.

- *How might my reactions to stress and loss be changed?* Are there alternative ways of responding? Could these toxic circumstances and relationships be removed from your life? If not, how can you balance them, honoring your own emotional needs first?

Give yourself permission to define your true needs. This is highly important wellness work. It is perfectly acceptable to find constructive and uplifting ways to meet these needs, regardless of what others may say or think. Give yourself that permission. Understand the message cancer has for you.

An Essential Thing to Do

Conduct a thorough and unflinching personal inventory. In your Wellness and Recovery Journal, complete this exercise:

1. High-stress event(s) that occurred in the year or two prior to diagnosis or recurrence included _____

_____

_____

2. My major emotional responses to these high-stress events were _____

_____

_____

3. I could have changed these circumstances by _____

_____

_____

4. I could have changed my emotional response by _____

_____

_____

Complete the inventory and then stop your wellness work for today. Carefully contemplate the implications of the important issues raised in this exercise. You may wish to revise your responses after a time of reflection.

#38

LIVE
NOW

Many people with a diagnosis of cancer needlessly pollute their lives by living in the past or in the future. Instead, I suggest our goal should be to live well with the only time we do have—this very precious present moment.

How many times have you heard yourself say, "If only I hadn't done such and such?" "If only I hadn't smoked." "If only I'd taken better care of myself." "If only . . ." "If only . . ." "If only . . ." We mire ourselves in the regrets of the past and miss the moment we have been given.

At other times we get caught in the fear of the future. "What if the cancer spreads?" "What if the chemo fails?" "What if . . ." "What if . . ." "What if . . ." Here we miss the present moment because we are consumed with what may happen in the future.

The answer: present-moment living. Live now. Live today. Live this hour. All of our regrets about the past, no matter how sincere, won't change history. All our worries about the future won't add even another minute to our lives. On the contrary, both fears and worries diminish our current moments.

Wellness and happiness are not completely dependent on your body's physical condition. High-level wellness is possible even with disability. Appreciate the fact that, even with cancer, you have life, here, now. Living each moment fully is the master secret to well-being.

Wellness has everything to do with the quality of our time; it's about this moment. Don't put off living a full life until you are physically "better." Now is the time! This is your moment!

"I was consumed with worry," said Brenda Barnes, a non-Hodgkin's lymphoma patient, "not just over my cancer, but about my entire life. My parents were divorced and I worried about my mother's emotional health. My dad traveled a lot and I worried about his airplanes crashing. What about my student loans that still hung over my head, unpaid for several years? Why couldn't I maintain a relationship with a man? Was I just an intractable failure in life? And then my illness, on top of it all."

Corwin Johnson was diagnosed with colon cancer at the age of fifty-six. "It (the cancer diagnosis) came two years after my injection molding business failed. All I could think of in those two years was what I should have done differently. If only I had not put so much emphasis on the new product line. Why didn't I see the downturn in the economy? Why did I extend so much credit to our number one customer? I should have announced shorter work weeks or layoffs much sooner. Why didn't I listen to the banker? How am I ever going to get out of debt? If only the family didn't have to suffer. Life is so unfair, I'm ruined."

Brenda and Corwin have a similar problem. Both are absolutely contaminating their present moments. Brenda's worries about the future assure her of enjoying little peace in this moment. Corwin's life is consumed by thoughts of self-judgment that imprison him in the past. Neither is living in the "now." Yet their only chance to capture true wellness is found in the now. What is required is a shift in thinking from what Corwin might have done in the past or what may happen to Brenda in the future, to what each can do right here, right now. What about you? Might similar shifts be required?

Our potential for knowing wellness depends on our ability to understand that the past does not equal the future. Living in the now frees us from an internal bondage that keeps us from following the wellness path.

The past is over. Regrets, remorse, and recrimination cannot touch us unless we allow them to remain in our lives. The future cannot harm us unless we create a future based on perceptions of fear, anger, and guilt. The only time that contains the power to change our lives is the present moment.

Just because you have cancer now does not predict, with certainty, that you will have it next year. Understand that truth. You have power in this moment that can change your life. Exercise that power—now!

An Essential Thing to Do

Each day, relinquish any thoughts or judgments that hold you to the past. Give up any fears that keep you from creating a healthy future. Pick one activity this day, this moment, that brings you pleasure, contentment, and happiness. Do it now! Know that the supply of these moments is limitless, there for the taking if you will only choose to do so. Here, in the present moment, you will find your wellness.

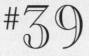

#39

Take
Time
to Play

How much time have you allowed yourself for play in the last week? If you answered "None," you are a member of a very large club. That's unfortunate. Living well requires play.

It's a common phenomenon. Many adults react negatively to the idea that we need to play. In fact, millions of people believe that grown-ups should not play. Somehow we think that playing is not the mature thing to do. Challenge this thinking. From this moment forward, I want you to understand that play is an important part of your "work" of wellness!

The need to honor our playful nature is very strong. Most of us just repress it. Don't. Give yourself permission to play, actually scheduling play time in your daily calendar if you must. I did. We must then treat that time carefully, assigning it the same importance and priority as other areas of life, such as work and family.

Sometimes we get fooled into thinking we are playing when we really are not. Eli Goldman, who was diagnosed with multiple myeloma, was also a member of a barbershop quartet. He thought his singing was play. Then Eli began to look at his "play" more closely. He soon realized his singing wasn't as much play as it was competition, a pressure to win contests, a pressure he did not need. Eli dropped out of the quartet and substituted kite making, in which the competition was strictly self-imposed. What a valuable lesson!

Analyze your own life. Have you noticed that you're never too tired to play? In fact, if you think you're tired, perhaps that is just the signal that you need more play. Play builds energy reserves; it is a major contributor to wellness.

God didn't create us just to work, work, and work. We were created for joy. So create some joy in your life. Consider this list of ten noncompetitive play activities:

1. Stroll on the beach.
2. Fly a kite.
3. Swim.
4. Ride a bike.
5. Draw a picture.
6. Write a poem.
7. Skip around the yard.
8. Sing.
9. Listen to music.
10. Take the scenic route.

An Essential Thing to Do

Make your own play list and record it in your Wellness and Recovery Journal. Now, I want you to stop reading. Put aside this book, right now, and go play for thirty minutes. Go! Have some fun. Do it! We'll continue our wellness work later.

#40

LAUGH
FOR
HEALING
POWER

Norman Cousins made many contributions to our understanding of the mind's role in mobilizing the body's healing processes. But none is so vividly remembered as his emphasis on laughter. In his 1981 book, *Anatomy of an Illness*, Cousins called laughter "internal jogging." Since that time, science has confirmed that even something as simple as a laugh or a smile carries with it a positive biochemical response.

The message is clear: lighten up! It will directly enhance your well-being. Just notice how relaxed you feel after laughing at a good story or watching a funny movie. It's wonderful!

Jack Abrams is a New York investment banker, successful, wealthy, the owner of a beautiful home in Westchester County, and the recipient of a metastatic prostate cancer diagnosis. "I thought, my God, I'm going to die. Cancer was the most god-awful threat I had ever faced." Jack received radiation treatment at a Manhattan medical center where he met Delmar, an older gentleman who always had a humorous story to share. Delmar had successfully completed the same treatment for prostate cancer some seven years earlier. Now he volunteers three days a week at the hospital. "My job," said Delmar, "is court jester!"

For most of us, seriousness is seen as an important virtue. "Gravitas" we call it. We tend to think that laughing or giggling is childish behavior and certainly not appropriate for adults. Jack used to subscribe to this thinking. "After all," he remarked, "investment banking is serious business. You have to be serious to be taken seriously."

Baloney! I observe way too many cancer patients going through life with this fearful, beaten, and downtrodden seriousness surrounding them. There is nothing inconsistent about being an adult and including laughter in your life. There is nothing wrong with being ill and pursuing a lighthearted approach to wellness. This is not some demented form of personal denial. Instead, it can be the opportunity to let the hidden child in you come out once in a while. Get in touch with that exuberant, vibrant part of yourself. Enjoy playing with your own children or grandchildren. Laugh at yourself and your seriousness.

Jack reflected, "Delmar taught me a lot about living. When I stopped being so serious, I started to get well."

An Essential Thing to Do

Go ahead. Rent that comedy DVD. Watch your favorite sitcom. Go to the local comedy club or a silly movie. Laugh! Let those positive biochemicals loose. It's healing.

#41

EVALUATE
YOUR
RELATIONSHIPS

Our relationships. We constantly interact with other people—a husband or wife, a friend or a lover, a child, a relative, a boss, a coworker, or an employee; the list of our relationships is endless. At times, our lives seem to center entirely on relationships. How we get along with the significant people in our lives seems to determine, to a large extent, the quality of life we have. Furthermore, the absence of relationships can cause much disharmony and deep dissatisfaction. Like it or not, relationships are central to our experience of life and even our experience of illness.

Cancer survivors invest time and energy in two-way relationships that nurture them. Survivors put relationships that are toxic "on hold." Patricia shared in a support group meeting what this meant to her. "I had to move out. It was difficult, particularly leaving my two children. But I knew it was what I needed at that time. And I stayed away for nearly three months."

Patricia married while in college. She went to work to support her husband and his education. Patricia was expecting her first child before her husband graduated from dental school. She never earned her degree, something her husband seemed to hold over her.

"He was always criticizing me," Patricia said. "And I would yell back, trying to defend myself from attack. I'd bring up times when he disappointed me. And he would counter with a litany of my shortcomings. It became a vicious cycle. So I got out of there."

Was a marriage gone askew partly responsible for Patricia's cervical cancer? I believe so. Toxic stress lowers our resistance. Sadly, Patricia's search for love led to an extramarital affair. The guilt became overwhelming, leading to clinical depression. Patricia came to believe the breach in her marriage was linked to her physical problems. After beginning her cancer treatment program, she finally began to look at the relationship with her husband.

Credit Patricia with wanting the relationship to work. With the help of a marriage counselor she was able to better understand her part in the ongoing battles. Patricia recognized her reactions and began to select other more measured responses to her husband's remarks. Today, Patricia and her husband are working on improving their relationship, and Patricia is cancer-free.

Here's a key insight you can use to your tremendous benefit. Our relationships with others often reflect the relationship we have with ourselves. Do you experience conflict with a coworker? Look within to understand the inner conflict you may carry. Does a child seem self-willed and impossible? Look within. Do you carry a belief that kids are willful and impossible?

Your self-perceptions are exceedingly powerful. They dramatically impact your relationships. And spiritually, even though we may have some changes of perception to make, it's the set of the heart that matters. If our hearts are in the right place—on the path of love, joy, and peace—our spiritual well-being is assured. All this takes is an internal search of our motives.

This internal search is our only real point of influence. When we evaluate relationships, the central task is to look within, discovering the truth: the only way to change another is to change ourselves first.

Be an encourager in all your relationships. Know that whatever you send out will always come back to you. Change and improve your relationships by sending out the love, joy, and peace that will help you heal. Truly, this is your point of power.

Do healed relationships always equate with healed bodies? I believe the two go together, but I can cite only anecdotal evidence. When we stop punishing ourselves and others for things that happened in the past, we are then free to move on to a life of wellness, a state of mind and spirit that often supports vast and rapid physical improvement.

An Essential Thing to Do

Conduct an inventory of the ten most important relationships in your life. Number a page in your Wellness and Recovery Journal from 1 through 10 and record the people's names. Did you realize these were the ten most important people in your life?

Highlight any relationships that need to be put on hold. Are there any that need improvement? Indicate those. What is one thing you could change that would improve each relationship?

Come back to this list often. Keep it current. Declare any "relationship war" to be over! Declare that you now live in joy and peace. Appreciate how important this work is to your achievement of wellness.

#42

GET
BEYOND
"WHY?"

It's the inevitable question cancer patients ask: "Why did this happen to me?"

The trouble with the "why?" question is that we seldom like the answers we are given. We fight them, not wanting to accept. Some think cancer is a lifestyle issue: "He smoked." That may be true for some but does not stand up to scrutiny for all cancer patients or even all smokers. Others say the "why?" is environmental: "We've polluted the planet. We're all getting sick." That may explain some cases, but why is it that other people exposed to the same carcinogens remain perfectly healthy?

Religion tries to answer the "Why me?" question. I've been told by well-meaning clergy that God was using cancer to punish my sins, to correct me for my eternal profit, to draw me closer to God, and to help me and my family members learn submission. Incredible!

When we ask "why?" we are often looking for someone or something to blame. "Why?" is another way of saying we are helpless and the situation is beyond our control. Some people blame others, some blame circumstances, some blame parents, some blame doctors, some blame the environment, and some blame God. Affixing blame does not help. It only creates helpless victims, something I trust by now you believe you are not.

The road to personal wellness starts when we stop asking "why?" and begin to consider the question, "Toward what end?" or "For what purpose?" Put another way, "How can I make this experience benefit myself, others, and the world?"

Literally thousands of the cancer survivors I have interviewed and surveyed speak of "God not being done with me quite yet." Could that be the case with you? Instead of asking, "Why me?" let's ask, "How can this illness best be used?" Then quiet yourself and listen. Let this idea settle deep in your spirit. It's the essence of getting beyond the "why?" of cancer.

An Essential Thing to Do

In your Wellness and Recovery Journal, start a new page with the heading "How can I make my experience of cancer beneficial?" Describe, in writing, how you believe cancer can help you and others. Continually add to this list as your insights deepen.

#43

PRACTICE
SELF-DISCIPLINE

Living a life based on maximizing your well-being requires living with values and behaviors that may be radically different from the ones you had before your illness. Some days, the work of wellness may not be the easiest or most convenient to practice. On a cold and rainy morning, it might be easier to stay in bed and forget the exercise. And instead of preparing a high-nutrition lunch, it might seem simpler to use the drive-through window of the nearest fast-food restaurant. Our intention to move toward wellness may seem strong, but too often our practices may not reflect that intent.

I encourage you to see yourself as self-disciplined. Wellness self-discipline includes thought and deed, intent and practice. This principle is equally valid whether you are facing a just-baked batch of chocolate-chip cookies, a dark cold morning of exercise, or an unforgivable person. Gentle, wholesome self-discipline is at the core of making wellness real in your life.

The issue is not whether we *can* choose wellness. It's whether we *see ourselves* choosing wellness. Remember, "The me I see is the me I'll be."

The practice of seeing yourself as self-disciplined leads to two very powerful life qualities: self-respect and freedom. When your walk matches your talk, when intent and action are one, you have a consistency in your life that is unshakable. You are grounded in a principle-oriented life experience, firm in the knowledge that all you are doing physically, emotionally, and spiritually is in your best interest.

Just for a moment, envision yourself as happily self-disciplined. Inner strength and self-respect flow from this position. The discipline to actually act on what is important to you leads to personal freedom; you are no longer bound by the traps of obsession, compulsion, and self-pity. This is a personal power at the highest level, a strong and quiet inner assurance that is one of the rewards of the wellness journey.

When I get up in the morning, the first thing I do is pull on my sweats and running shoes. No excuses. I discipline myself to exercise.

Diet was a wellness discipline that challenged me. I loved sweets, especially pastries. Today, I simply do not allow myself to indulge. I deserve better nutrition. Discipline.

Meditation—when do I have time to fit this into a busy schedule? Yet I do, twice each day. Dicipline. My times of meditation result in a clearer perspective on the day, a perspective that I refuse to live without.

The same is true for developing a purpose/play balance, nurturing my relationships, and honoring my spiritual needs. Each important area of my life requires a consistent disciplined practice in order for me to know its potential. I see you doing something very similar. It starts with seeing yourself as self-disciplined and actually doing the work of wellness.

"But that's no fun," protested Manuel Morales, a big, burly mechanical engineer with kidney cancer. He was attending one of our workshops in San Antonio. "You're right," I responded, "It's better than fun. It's freedom—freedom from all that hurts us."

Self-discipline. The issue becomes which habits we will choose in our lives. Choose a positive addiction. Decide to discipline yourself to choose the habits of wellness. The result is self-respect and freedom.

An Essential Thing to Do

Match your walk with your talk, your actions with your best intentions. Choose one area—perhaps diet or exercise—and make that your focus today. For example, pick one day and excel at maximizing your nutrition. Then choose another area for focus for the next day. And another the next. Feel your self-respect skyrocket. Congratulate yourself. Bask in the personal power and freedom this discipline brings to you.

#44

Choose
Your
Emotional
Style

What is your dominant style of expressing emotion? Is it suppression, where you constantly restrain yourself from venting real feelings; or overreaction, where you are too exuberant or fly into inappropriate rage; or denial, where you tend to push feelings out of your consciousness?

If you have read this book to this point, you now know that emotions have a central role in wellness. Two emotional styles concern me most: fear that is denied and hostility that is either suppressed or overexpressed. Our goal here is to become a skilled observer of our emotional reactions and learn the ability to choose appropriate responses.

You have the right to feel any emotion. Any and every emotion you feel is perfectly acceptable. We're human; we feel. In a real sense, we are emotionally driven creatures. One moment we're angry, the next moment we're down. We're happy and we laugh. The next moment we're fearful of some loss. I've observed that people tend to repeatedly experience four basic emotions: mad, sad, glad, and e'gad—anger, depression, happiness, and fear. All of them are acceptable.

To experience an emotion, and recognize that any emotion is acceptable, is one level of understanding. But the healthful processing of those emotions is quite another. It's here we typically find trouble.

You have tremendous power over your emotions. It's the power of choice. Health-enhancing emotional processing is summarized by the phrase *review, release, and renew.*

Review the emotion. The most damaging mistake we make in emotional expression is to attach too high a priority on either burying or venting the feeling. Instead, start by observing the emotion. Review it. Understand it. That's half the challenge.

Then release the emotion. Get rid of the anger, the sadness, the fear. It's perfectly acceptable to feel the way you feel. It's your emotion and you own it. But then release it in a nonhostile way, without being coy, subtle, or vague. Think or say, "I'm upset but it's only my emotions. It's over and done. Life goes on." Release.

Then renew. Think and say, "I can choose my emotions. My emotions do not choose me." You replace it. Consciously, cognitively, you choose a more productive, more loving, more spiritual emotional response.

This process is so very powerful. For example, my personal emotional challenge is effectively processing anger, one of the most highly charged emotions. My anger is generally short-lived, a negative emotion over a single event. When I'm functioning at my best, I'll review it: "There's my anger. I recognize it. It's starting to boil my water." Then I'll release it: "Anger. Go away. I become upset when you're around." I express it, without malice. I release it.

The trouble comes when I don't renew, when I fail to consciously replace that anger with love, or at least compassion. When I allow anger to continue to control my responses, I am plagued by chronic anger that wears a mask. It appears to be anger but it is actually unresolved hostility—toxic emotions and feelings to which I cling. It's like walking through a field that is filled with landmines. The slightest nudge and an explosion erupts.

One of the demands of living well is to no longer cling to negative emotions. We cling with coping styles of denial, suppression,
and overreaction. Not until we review, release, and honestly
renew can we become masters of our emotions.

You also have this power. Renewal is actually very simple. For
me it comes when I focus my attention on what actually provoked
me. If I will just reflect on the event, I will often discover that I
perceived the provoker—be it a person, event, or condition—
with fear. I was the one who was fearful that my person, property,
or pride was under attack.

This is a profound discovery of the highest importance, one
that affects us on every level of our lives. It's fear we are dealing
with, actually our perception of fear, something that is under our
control. Now we can review and release that fear, and verbalize it.
"This diagnosis scares me." Or, "Doctor, I reject that prognosis."

Then, and only then, can we transcend emotionally. We renew;
we consciously choose a more powerful and productive emotion.
"I choose to be hopeful—anyway."

That's why it is so important that we become keenly aware of
our emotional style. Simply observing the situations that trigger
our emotions allows us to rethink our perception that we are
under siege. Instead of perceiving fear, we can now understand
the situation in the light of love, or at least compassion. This is a
new and miraculous emotional response, one that immediately
begins to dissolve resentments and helps immensely in our
healing.

Make it your priority to become a keen observer of your own
emotions. Review, release, and renew. It is the secret to emotional
well-being.

An Essential Thing to Do

Become an objective observer over the next week. When an
upsetting event occurs, record the event in your Wellness and
Recovery Journal. Then record your emotional response based on
one of three categories: denial—"I denied that there was any

problem"; suppression—"I suppressed my emotions when I really wanted to tell them off"; or overreaction—"I went crazy and overreacted, way out of proportion to the whole event."

Then practice the three Rs: review, release, and renew. You'll become a skilled observer of your own emotional stance toward life. Reactions and emotions that were once automatic will now come under your control. Through it all, you will achieve new levels of well-being.

THE SEVENTH STEP: NURTURE YOUR SPIRIT

I trust you have been following and implementing the steps in this book. If so, you are well on your way to triumph over cancer.

Many cancer survivors go even further, reaching for higher levels of well-being in all areas of their lives.

"I see it [cancer] as a gift," said singer Olivia Newton-John about her journey through breast cancer. "I know it sounds strange. But I don't think I would have grown in the areas I did without this experience."

Seek the gift in cancer. It's there. Join me now in continuing this search.

#45

SEE
LIFE
THROUGH
SPIRITUAL
EYES

What do you see when you look at your life? Do you see a body riddled with disease, dreams hopelessly derailed, a family frightened, and life lived in despair?

Or can you see a precious moment, a special instant in space and time where mind and spirit are ill only if you allow it? Can you see the beauty and grace, even the perfection, in your life without coloring those qualities with the pain of cancer?

Peter Halters was a forty-year-old father who developed pancreatic cancer. It was a difficult battle, especially since he wanted so very much to live. His valiant efforts were an inspiration to many people. During one of our telephone sessions, Peter remarked, "I think the spiritual part began to make sense last night. We were at the dinner table, the whole family. And I saw something different. It really stuck with me."

"What do you mean?" I asked.

"Well, before last night, I always saw the obvious at the dinner table: the chicken, the salad, and the mashed potatoes. I'd see my wife, looking tired and worried like she was always running behind schedule. And the kids with a thousand stories of things happening at school. That was what was in front of me. That's what I saw.

"But last night I saw from my heart," continued Peter, struggling to hold back tears. "I looked around that table and saw something quite different. For the first time, I was able to see this precious moment where the minds, bodies, and souls of our family were gathered together to break bread and be nourished. There was so much more there than just the food. There were lives filled with potential for good. We were there to help each other, to love and care for each other."

Peter paused as he relived that special moment in his mind. "Then the children got into an argument with their mother. But instead of driving me up the wall, this conflict was somehow different. Or at least I saw it differently. It seemed to be a natural expression of love toward each other, a way of saying, 'I care.'"

Peter was looking through spiritual eyes. Spiritual eyes allow us to see the value of what is simple and readily available in our lives in spite of the circumstances in which we may find ourselves.

"I awoke from my surgery," said Pontea Kamal, "and there in my room was my husband. He was holding our little daughter, propping her up on the hospital bed. And she was squeezing my finger. Her big dark eyes looked at me, and she smiled as she said, 'I love you, Mommy.' It was such a precious moment. Now, since my cancer, I see so much deeper into life."

Make a commitment. Join me in no longer dwelling on what is wrong and taking inventory of what is missing. Let's put our focus on all that is right, all that we have. And we have a lot.

This level of awareness brings a vastly different experience of cancer and of life. Embrace this consciousness. There are miraculous moments in your life right now—each and every day. See them.

An Essential Thing to Do

Stop. Take a few minutes to see life in this new, more spiritual light. Ask yourself, "What do my countless blessings really mean to me?" This new awareness may contribute more toward your well-being than the most potent medicine.

#46

VALUE
PERSONAL
SPIRITUAL
GROWTH

Too many people equate victory over cancer with a doctor's report that says, "This patient is clinically free of cancer." I understand that desire, I share that desire, and, in fact, my records state exactly that. I wish you the same. But that is not the most important part of the journey through cancer.

Please read carefully. Consider these next words deeply. For the person who opens his or her mind and spirit, the cancer experience evolves into a transcendent spiritual journey. The real triumph over cancer is realized in the nurturing of personal spiritual growth.

Some people say, "Greg, I'll settle for a cure. Just get my life back to normal." Don't settle for that! You don't want things to get back to normal. After your experience with cancer, things will never be the same again. You want a new and better life. That life comes in the form of a new spiritual walk.

Cancer has pounded you with a million hammer blows. But you have the last word as to how those blows will shape you. William James, the distinguished psychologist and philosopher, declared that his generation's most important discovery was that human beings, by changing their inner attitudes of mind, could change the outer aspects of their lives.

I see you changing in that way, using the hammer blows of cancer to change your inner state of spirit. By making personal spiritual growth our aim, the most important discovery will be to use the experience of cancer to shape us into wonderfully different people. Indeed, cancer can reshape our attitudes, soften our spirits, and transform our lives.

It's personal spiritual growth we seek. You have those seeds of well-being inside you. But it's up to you to believe and act on them.

Think of personal spiritual growth as the natural and logical extension of your wellness journey. The steps are simple. You are going to make a decision to do all possible to get well again. You are going to devote time and energy to understanding your treatment options, to improving your diet, to daily exercise, to making positive beliefs and attitudes real in your life, and to nurturing your most important relationships.

Then, in a very seamless progression, you'll explore and develop your own practices of gratitude, forgiveness, unconditional love, and more. It's the spiritual part of the wellness journey.

Are you ready? It's the most important part of the trip.

Cynicism has no place here. You cannot climb up the spiritual mountain by thinking downhill thoughts. If you feel that life is filled with despair, that it is gloomy and hopeless, and that spiritual growth is impossible for you, it is because you are gloomy and hopeless. You must change your inner world, which will in turn change your outer world.

Powerful healing awaits you. Associate with people who are walking the spiritual path. Your spiritual journey can be advanced by meeting and mingling with those who have a spiritual vision. Be inspired by our great spiritual ancestors from all the ages.

And pray. Be still and prayerfully listen to God. Don't beg or plead. Pray, "Thy will be done." Then listen. And act.

Please, don't limit God's infinite possibilities by imposing your conditions for wellness. God can use you even with cancer. Be open to that spiritual experience. Remember, with God, all things are possible.

An Essential Thing to Do

In your Wellness and Recovery Journal, record one spiritual quality that you would like to make vivid and real in your life. Start by making a commitment to practice that quality for just one hour. Then extend the time. Keep this as your central goal. Pray and listen for guidance. Opportunities for practice will present themselves every moment of the day. Seize them.

#47

MAKE
FORGIVENESS
A HABIT

Do you want to free all your energy to heal? Forgive! Let go! Release!

Forgiveness is wellness work that brings with it huge rewards. Forgiveness links our newfound awareness of the healing dynamics with our awakened understanding of our emotional style. The promised benefit of this linkage is the emotional and spiritual peace and serenity we need for healing.

This is a big promise. Forgiveness can deliver.

I believe forgiveness, when it actually becomes a way of thinking and living, is the single most powerful key to wellness. Forgiveness is a trusted technique by which our thoughts and perceptions are changed, transforming the harmful effects of toxic emotions into the healing reality of compassion, even love. Forgiveness allows us to switch our focus from fear to love; it helps us change what can be changed and allows us to make peace with the rest—a profound dimension of healing.

Opportunities to learn and practice forgiveness are everywhere. The obvious teachers of forgiveness come in the form of people, most often individuals who antagonize us, the ones whom we can't stand to be around.

But more important than forgiving others is teaching ourselves to be self-forgiving. It all starts with our own power and control.

Let's be honest; we hold much resentment and shame against ourselves; we don't let go easily. In the quiet moments we judge ourselves harshly: "I'm so stupid. I'm fat. I'm ugly. I'm not worthy. I probably deserve this illness." The list is without end.

Now, with cancer, like never before, this is the moment to release that self-condemnation. The only way is through self-forgiveness.

Let go. I observe so many cancer patients carrying self-concepts of unworthiness. These are false and deadly beliefs. Yes, we may have done something undesirable, but that is our behavior and does not equate with being an unworthy person. Release those feelings of unworthiness.

A young single mother shared, "I was a drug addict and a prostitute. Now cancer. But I think I deserve it. God is punishing me."

"No," I responded. "Absolutely not! Release those beliefs. They are serving only to condemn you to a life of disease. Forgive yourself. Forgive others. Ask God to forgive you. Release it all."

There's more. Beyond ourselves, our perceptions of others can also create a battleground of emotional turmoil. It is so easy to judge others. Judgmental behavior tears at the fabric of relationships and kindles the fires of resentment. Cancer is, among other things, an opportunity to learn and practice the difference between acceptance and approval, to transcend judgment.

I urge you to practice acceptance. A man with metastatic prostate cancer came to our offices and soon began to tell the tale of his son who was gay. There was so much strife between the two—fights, accusations, condemnation. The son left for college and never returned home. For over six years, the two hardly spoke. It weighed so heavily on the father. Then he got his cancer diagnosis.

"I knew that forgiveness and reconciliation were central to my getting well again," said the man. "I finally reached my son on the phone and said I would like to see him. When we met, the first thing I promised was to never again mention his lifestyle. I made a decision to release it all—his lifestyle and my health—to God."

Forgive. Let go. Release. Yes, forgiveness is *the* answer. All of us have imperfect natures. All of us exhibit behaviors that don't match our potential. Forgiveness allows us to accept imperfection without having to approve of it. Have you noticed? Not everything in life meets your expectations. But we can find peace through acceptance. Yes, we still distinguish right from wrong. But forgiving ourselves and others is at the heart of practicing acceptance. Let go.

Join me. Let's begin to make the practice of forgiveness a habit. Forgiveness is experienced on two levels. The first is the most obvious. There is an event: Someone is wronged or we perceive an attack. That behavior needs to be forgiven. When we can say, "I forgive myself for _____," or "I forgive _____ (another) for _____," then we have embarked upon the forgiveness journey.

The second level of forgiveness changes our perception of what happened. Yes, an event occurred. But the real problem starts when we begin to judge what happened, when we label ourselves or the other person as bad, hurtful, mean, stupid, or with some other less-than-kind attribute. We perceived the event as unfavorable; the event didn't meet our approval. We judge, even condemn, the people involved.

The alternative? Acceptance. Accept ourselves. Accept others. Accept that events happen. Accept that life is often far from our glittering ideals. Forgive and accept. This is a far better way to live.

People who are, or believe themselves to be, near death often come to the realization that forgiveness heals. Feuds, differences, and deep hurts suddenly seem less important at this time. I can understand. I had to learn this lesson myself. Literally thousands of patients share similar stories.

Marilyn Ellis, in the middle of a battle with ovarian cancer, felt terribly ill at ease when her mother and father visited. Marilyn and her mother would make noble efforts to get along with each other, but they seldom fully succeeded. Old patterns of attack and defense were constantly cropping up between them. Child care, cooking, homemaking, religion—the particulars didn't seem to matter. Her mother wanted a more conservative daughter. Marilyn wanted a more enlightened mother.

"It was driving me crazy," said Marilyn. "During her last visit, I was ready to throw her out. But then it occurred to me, God isn't looking at my mother and thinking, 'Mildred is so impossible.' How could I pretend to want to get along with my mother if I was so consumed by my judgment of her errors? I had to practice acceptance and get off my fixation with approval.

"So I said to myself, 'I'll try this for an afternoon. I'll focus on acceptance and give up approval.' From that moment, the situation and the relationship started to shift. As I was more accepting of her, she became more accepting of me. We're a long way from best buddies," conceded Marilyn, "but there is a growing bond between us."

Maybe you struggle with hostility and resentment. If so, forgive. The amazing payoff of forgiveness is that so many people do get well after letting go. Lives are certainly made better; many are made longer. But it strikes me that if one is willing to forgive during the last moments of life, why not do it earlier? Like right now?

How often do we need to forgive? Always. Don't drag the memories of past hurts and mistakes into your present moments. Nothing from the past is important enough to allow it to pollute our present. Forgive. Let go of judgment. Become a shining example of compassion. You deserve it. You'll change your life—forever!

An Essential Thing to Do

Choose just one hurt or mistake and forgive everyone concerned with it. Say out loud, "(Name), I totally and completely forgive you. I release you to the care of God. I affirm your highest good." Mean it. Now feel the warmth of forgiveness. Choose to forgive one person each day.

#48

EXUDE GRATITUDE

What is the least-healthy spiritual habit, the one that causes disease of every kind? It's ingratitude—the lack of thankfulness, our inadequate appreciation for all the blessings we enjoy.

Have you expressed your thankfulness today? We all have so many blessings to appreciate every day of our lives. But most of us overlook them. The conscious practice of being grateful is central to the healing process.

Even with cancer, even in the middle of a difficult treatment cycle, even in your darkest and most fearful hours, be thankful for all you do have. For life, for love, for family, for friends, for the awesome beauty of nature, for the presence of God, for all these things and more, be thankful.

Why do I feel so strongly about gratitude's healing power? It's because I have seen gratitude bring more significant and rapid improvements to the lives of cancer patients than any other single action. Thousands of survivors are convinced that there is a physiological correlative to gratitude, and their bodies respond. I agree.

Be grateful. If you wish to cultivate a deeper attitude of gratitude, I suggest you begin to see yourself as a guest who is only visiting here on earth. All that you have is not really yours; it is a gracious gift from your host. You are privileged to enjoy the gifts of friends and family, home and transportation, food and recreation, vocation and service, during your stay. Even your health, no matter what the state, is another of those gifts.

Jill Phillips lay near death in a small rural Nebraska hospital after being told she was "filled" with cancer and that it was inoperable. Mired in despair and self-pity, she could see nothing for which she could be thankful. "I was divorced, my two children were grown and lived in different parts of the country. I hated my dead-end job. My life seemed miserable.

"But one night I looked out of my hospital window to see a deep, dark sky that was filled with stars. I shut off all the lights in my room and just gazed at the sky for what must have been hours. I started to ask a lot of questions: 'What is this huge universe about? What is my place in it? Why am I sick?' I can't say I got a lot of answers. But I did get a different perspective.

"I became thankful," continued Jill, "grateful just for being a part of this huge and wonderful world. I realized that in my fifty-plus years, I had been able to experience so much. The marvel of giving birth to two other lives—what a miracle! The beauty of the country, where I feel such strong roots; I was so grateful to live here rather than in a city. The deep friendship I had with my sister—I was so thankful for her love. That night at the window changed my whole perspective on my problems."

Like Jill, we too can capture true well-being when we choose gratitude. But so many roadblocks on the cancer journey seem to detour us, to mire us in ruts of ingratitude and self-pity. We're so busy with appointments and treatments, discomfort and despair, fear and pain, that we lose our perspective. We tend to look at the cancer journey as a long and twisted path, filled with potholes. There seems to be nothing for which we can be thankful. This is faulty and self-destructive thinking.

Every day start saying aloud, "I am so grateful for all I have been given, even my next breath." Exude gratitude. It transforms the very experience of illness and of life. I implore you, see beyond the day-to-day experiences that seem so all-consuming. Treasure the wonder of life. Become aware of your "guest status" in this brief moment in time and space. Be thankful. Exude gratitude. It heals.

An Essential Thing to Do

It's time for another page in your Wellness and Recovery Journal. Complete the following sentence:

I am so happy and grateful now that _____.

Express your gratitude—every hour of every day.

49

PRACTICE
UNCONDITIONAL
LOVING

Loving heals. Even though there may be times when we are lost in the abyss of our physical maladies or buried in the agony of our emotional awfulizing, with each moment comes a new opportunity to choose loving. This is a decision that truly heals.

I prefer the word *loving* over *love*. It denotes the action necessary to bring the idea of love to life. Love is not loving until it is released, until it is intentionally given.

Loving without conditions is an intentional choice we make to determine what is coming *through* us rather than what is coming *to* us. The choice to love means we don't have to wait for the medical test results, the doctor's assurances, the elusive remission, or the hoped-for cure. We can choose to love now, this moment. And the next moment. And the next. We always have this power of choice, regardless of the circumstances. This choice heals.

Consider this perspective. The crippling fears surrounding cancer are actually the absence of love. The fear is like darkness that is merely the absence of light. You don't solve a problem of darkness by yelling at it or trying to strike at it. If you want to get rid of the darkness, you turn on a light.

So it is with fear. You don't fight it. You replace fear with love.

This is a profound and radical call, not some live-with-loving-feelings suggestion. Loving is more than a thin veneer. Loving is an act of heroism and courage of the highest order. You should not seek or even expect accolades. Unconditional loving is not a decision surrounded by pomp and circumstance. Most often it has to do with small choices. "How do I choose to respond to this person?" "How might I focus on the positive?" "How can I best help another person?" "How can I best love myself?"

By most standards, the conditions and circumstances of cancer do not inspire loving. Taken by themselves, the conditions may elicit despair; the cancer journey has many such moments. But we can take the loving action anyway! Invariably, the result is a renewed sense of hope that results in a strong biochemical "live" signal to body, mind, and spirit.

Loving starts with self-loving. You can hope to know wellness only from a position of personal emotional and spiritual strength. Self-loving is the wellspring of this vital force. Affirm your great value; cancer does not detract from your self-worth. Self-loving is the root of recovery for thousands of patients.

Does loving seem too difficult a task? Does your mind say that you can never be at peace until the cancer is gone? Do you feel that a total and complete physical cure is the only acceptable answer? Does it seem impossible to love with the sword of cancer balancing precariously over your head?

Love anyway. Focus on the love that comes *through* you and direct it to others. For if you love, you will be well.

Loving is the first and last word in healing, the great balm that quiets distress, the only real "magic bullet" against cancer, and the strongest vaccine to combat malignancy.

Our greatest enemy is not disease but despair. Unconditional loving is the healer.

An Essential Thing to Do

It is decision time. Decide to practice unconditional loving for the next hour. And the next hour, and the next. You will know healing—something far greater than a cure.

#50

SHARE THIS HOPE

Now that you've invested time reading this book and following at least some of the steps, you're aware that there is much you can do to improve your well-being. Your choices and actions really do make an enormous difference. In partnership with your medical team, you are on the pathway to healing.

But most people don't know these powerful truths. Or if they do, they have only a vague acquaintance with the strategies, not a working knowledge. They deserve more.

Share this hope with others who have been diagnosed with cancer. Discuss these ideas. Encourage one another. Make it your new priority to walk the path of wellness with someone else. This has the cumulative effect of helping yourself while helping another.

I invite you to contact us. We have a free e-newsletter for you, plus a variety of helpful wellness resources. Believe it: you have a caring partner in your journey.

Cancer Recovery Foundation International
www.cancerrecovery.org

Part Three

Essential Guides for the Journey

Guide 1:
Nutrition as
Medicine

The Vitamin D Promise

Beyond common skin cancer, and at current rates, one in two men and one in three women will personally be diagnosed with a major cancer in their lifetime. Breast cancer will account for the most common diagnosis among women. Prostate cancer will account for the most common diagnosis among men.

Here is the good news: excellent research indicates we can now prevent nearly 80 percent of all breast cancers. Observational research indicates that we may be able to prevent a substantial portion of all prostate cancers. Plus credible research points to the potential of preventing a significant number of other cancers. That's prevent—not early detection or early intervention, but prevention! That is a huge promise. It's real. It's vitamin D.

If you have followed the nutritional supplement field, you know I am required by law to say these statements have not been evaluated by the U.S. Food and Drug Administration. Further, I am required to note that vitamin D supplements are not intended to diagnose, treat, cure, or prevent any disease. But what I can say is to do the research and decide for yourself. Here are the facts:

A Basic Understanding

It all starts naturally with our own body's ability to manufacture vitamin D.

Natural production of vitamin D_3 cholecalciferol (pronounced koh•luh•kal•SIF•uh•rawl) in the skin is the single most important fact every person should know about vitamin D—a fact that has profound implications for the human condition. Technically not a vitamin, vitamin D is actually a hormone that interacts with over 2,000 genes, about 10 percent of the human genome. Extensive research has implicated vitamin D deficiency as a major factor in the pathology of at least fourteen varieties of cancer, most notably breast and prostate cancer, as well as a variety of other diseases.

Please understand that vitamin D is something we all need but something nearly all of us lack in adequate amounts. The deficiency is affecting our health.

The Science

Since 2005, cancer has become the leading cause of death for people under the age of eighty-five in America. Cancer now accounts for nearly one in every four deaths in the United States each year. It has also become the single leading cause of death worldwide. But scientific studies suggest that about three fourths of those cancer deaths could be avoided! Statistical analysis shows that two thirds of the deaths that occurred in 2010 alone, for example, were related to lifestyle choices such as tobacco use, obesity, physical inactivity, and poor nutrition and therefore could be prevented.

Enter vitamin D. Excellent science shows that an adequate level of vitamin D hinders inappropriate cell division and metastasis, decreases blood vessel formation around tumors, and regulates proteins that influence tumor growth. An adequate level of vitamin D also enhances the immune system's ability to fight cancer as well as promote the efficacy of several chemotherapeutic medicines.

In some of the most impressive research ever, studies conducted at the Creighton University School of Medicine in Nebraska have revealed that supplementing with vitamin D and calcium can reduce the risk of breast cancer by an astonishing 77 percent. This research provides strong new evidence that vitamin D is the single most effective preventative against breast cancer, far outpacing the benefits of any cancer drug known to modern science.

The four-year, randomized study followed 1,179 healthy, postmenopausal women from rural eastern Nebraska. Participants taking calcium, as well as a quantity of vitamin D_3 nearly three times the U.S. government's Recommended Daily Amount (RDA) for middle-age adults, showed a dramatic 60 percent or greater reduction in cancer risk than women who did not get the vitamin.

The results of the study, conducted between 2000 and 2005, were reported in the June 8, 2010, online edition of the *American Journal of Clinical Nutrition*.

"The findings are very exciting. They confirm what a number of vitamin D proponents have suspected for some time but that, until now, have not been substantiated through clinical trial," said principal investigator Joan Lappe, Ph.D., R.N., Creighton Professor of Medicine and holder of the Criss/Beirne Endowed Chair in the School of Nursing. "Vitamin D is a critical tool in fighting cancer as well as many other diseases."

Research participants were all fifty-five years and older and free of known cancers for at least ten years prior to entering the Creighton study. Subjects were randomly assigned to take daily dosages of 1,400 to 1,500 mg supplemental calcium, the calcium plus 1,100 IU of vitamin D, or placebos. The National Institutes of Health funded the study.

Over the course of four years, women in the calcium/vitamin D_3 group experienced a 60 percent decrease in their cancer risk than the group taking placebos.

On the premise that some women entered the study with undiagnosed cancers, researchers then eliminated the first-year results and looked at the last three years of the study. When they did that, the results became even more dramatic, with the calcium/vitamin D_3 group showing a startling 77 percent cancer risk reduction.

Please grasp the stunning implications of this study. Over four years, the group receiving the calcium and vitamin D supplements showed a 60 percent decrease in cancer. Considering just the last three years of the study reveals an impressive 77 percent reduction in cancer attributable solely to vitamin D supplementation.

These astonishing results were achieved on what many nutritionists consider to be a low dose of vitamin D. Exposure to sunlight, which creates even more vitamin D in the body, was not tested or considered. Plus the quality of the calcium supplements was likely not as high as it could have been. It was calcium carbonate and not high-grade calcium malate or aspartate.

Beyond this groundbreaking study, additional research demonstrates vitamin D to be an effective cancer preventative, particularly for breast cancer and prostate cancer. Numerous studies have shown an inverse correlation between breast cancer mortality and vitamin D levels—when vitamin D levels are low, cancer deaths are relatively high; when vitamin D levels are high, cancer deaths are relatively low. Today, over 1,900 scientific studies link vitamin D deficiency with various cancers.

But the cancer community has been reluctant, exceedingly slow to respond. Now I am asking you to study the evidence and decide for yourself. As you study, please consider the opinion of the experts, esteemed professionals in vitamin D research:

Cedric Garland, D.P.H., Adjunct Professor, Family & Preventive Medicine, Cancer Prevention & Control Program at the University of California at San Diego, states, "Breast cancer is a disease so directly related to vitamin D deficiency that a woman's risk of contracting the disease can be 'virtually eradicated' by elevating her vitamin D status to what scientists consider to be natural blood levels."

Dr. Michael F. Holick, Ph.D., M.D., and author of *The Vitamin D Solution*, reports that there is an incredible potential opportunity to prevent cancer simply by increasing the supply of vitamin D in the body through supplements. "As early as 1941, it was observed that people living at higher latitude were at higher risk of dying of cancer. In the 1980s, research revealed that living at higher latitude and being at higher risk of vitamin D deficiency increased risk of developing and dying of cancers of the colon, rectum, prostate, breast, and ovary. More recently, vitamin D deficiency has been associated with increased risk of developing many other cancers, including cancer of the esophagus and pancreas and leukemia. Participants in the Women's Health Initiative that evaluated the effect of calcium and vitamin D on risk of developing colorectal cancer revealed that women who were vitamin D deficient and followed for eight years had a 253 percent increased risk of developing colorectal cancer."

Anthony Norman, Ph.D., Professor of Biochemistry and Biomedical Sciences at the University of California at Riverside, states that the majority of scientists believe that the currently recommended daily intake of vitamin D (between 200 IU and 600 IU) is not enough. "There is a wide consensus among scientists that the relative daily intake of vitamin D should be increased to 2,000 to 4,000 IU for most adults."

Tracey O'Connor, M.D., an oncologist at Roswell Park Cancer Institute in Buffalo, New York, states she is now having all her patients supplement with vitamin D. Since vitamin D carries no risk unless taken at enormously high amounts, it can only benefit those who are already healthy by preventing disease, as well as those who are sick. Those with debilitating diseases have been found to be the most deficient in vitamin D, indicating a clear correlation between deficiency and the onset of disease. For example, Dr. O'Connor points out that among women with breast cancer, about 80 percent are vitamin D deficient.

An Opportunity Missed

A wide range of vitamin D experts, including the Cancer Recovery Foundation, believed the opportunity for a breakthrough might be possible when the governments of Canada and the United States commissioned an Institute of Medicine (IOM) review on vitamin D recommendations. After three years of study, the Institute's Food and Nutrition Board issued a report on November 30, 2010, saying it has revised its recommendations made thirteen years previously on dietary reference intakes for vitamin D and calcium for Americans and Canadians.

The committee, consisting of more than a dozen panelists, recommended that most Americans and Canadians up to age seventy need no more than 600 IU of vitamin D per day to maintain health. It also stated that those seventy-one and older may need as much as 800 IU.

The Food and Nutrition Board claimed in its news release that it reviewed nearly 1,000 published studies and testimony from scientists. It said many studies yielded conflicting and mixed results on the effects of vitamin D on many important health conditions including cancer, heart disease, autoimmune diseases, and diabetes, among others. The report concluded that no solid evidence suggests that higher than the recommended dietary reference intakes are needed.

The report was a huge disappointment to the hundreds of us dedicated to the task of actually preventing cancer. Cancer Recovery Foundation responded to the new recommendations in a news release stating that, "According to scientific studies, right now 70 percent of European-Americans and 97 percent of African-Americans are vitamin D deficient. And the evidence is overwhelming that vitamin D deficiency is directly linked to fourteen different cancers, mostly prominently breast and prostate cancer."

The IOM's report ignored research showing that in order to maintain adequate vitamin D levels, much higher doses of vitamin D must be consumed. Excellent research exists to support this position. Unfortunately, of the panelists included in the IOM recommendation, only a few had experience in vitamin D research. Even worse, the panel suppressed the findings of some of the world's most prominent vitamin D scientists, including our esteemed friends Cedric Garland, Michael Holick, and Anthony Norman.

Dr. John Cannell, M.D., a vitamin D expert and director of the Vitamin D Council, pointed out that the IOM's vitamin D recommendation that a baby and a pregnant woman need the same amount of vitamin D did not make any sense. He said his organization pressed the IOM to release the comments on vitamin D and health from fourteen vitamin D experts.

Cancer Recovery Foundation joined him with an online petition asking Harvey Fineberg, M.D., Ph.D., President of the Institute of Medicine, to include the testimony of these esteemed scientists. Thereafter, we filed a Freedom of Information request with the Institute of Medicine. Sadly, there has been no response.

In a follow-up statement, the Food and Nutrition Board suggested that without "solid" evidence, it is risky to recommend high intake of vitamin D. It cited vitamin E as an example to suggest that high intake of vitamin D could lead to toxicity issues.

That may sound convincing to some people. But at the sunniest time of a summer day, exposure of the face and arms to the sun for fifteen to twenty minutes is known to make a person more than 10,000 units of vitamin D. And there is no toxicity issue in such a natural dose.

The latitude at which you live and your ancestry influence your body's ability to convert sunlight into vitamin D. People with dark skin have more difficulty making the vitamin. Persons living at latitudes north of the 36th parallel cannot obtain adequate levels of vitamin D naturally during the winter months because of the sun's angle.

The research is convincing to all but the most skeptical scientists. Just some of the overwhelming evidence includes:

- Sunlight triggers the formation of vitamin D_3 in the skin, which is activated by the liver and kidneys into a hormone. This activated form of vitamin D supports "cellular differentiation," essentially the opposite of cancer.
- Vitamin D_3 has been repeatedly shown to inhibit the growth of malignant melanoma, breast cancer, leukemia, and mammary tumors in laboratory animals.
- Even synthetic vitamin D–like molecules have prevented the equivalent of breast cancer in laboratory animals.
- Vitamin D_3 has also been shown to inhibit angiogenesis, the growth of new blood vessels that permit the spread of cancer cells through the body.

For decades we have known of the evidence that women over fifty years of age who skimp on foods rich in vitamin D are more likely to develop breast cancer. The late Frank Garland, Ph.D., brother of Cedric, who also conducted vitamin D research at the University of California at San Diego, especially noted the anticancer protection of fish because fatty fish is packed with vitamin D.

Saint George's, University of London, previously known as Saint George's Hospital Medical School, found local production of vitamin D in breast tissue reduces the risk for breast cancer. For women with low breast tissue levels of vitamin D, the risk for breast cancer rose by a staggering 354 percent. This study even suggested women might wish to sunbathe with breast tissue exposed to enhance local vitamin D production.

Dr. Edward Giovannucci, Professor of Nutrition and Epidemiology at Harvard School of Public Health in Boston, Massachusetts, wrote his support of the Cancer Recovery Group recommendations:

Because most people do not get adequate vitamin D in typical diets, and because of the potential downsides of excessive sun exposure, most people may benefit from vitamin D supplements. Several groups are at risk for vitamin D deficiency or less-than-adequate intakes—in particular, the elderly, dark-skinned individuals, obese individuals, and those who avoid the sun. For those at a higher risk of vitamin D deficiency, a larger daily supplement dose, on the order of 3,000 to 4,000 IU, may be required to achieve adequate blood levels which in my opinion are in the range of 30–40 ng/mL based on current knowledge.

John H. White, Ph.D., Professor, Departments of Physiology and Medicine at McGill University, Montreal, Canada, concurred:

There is now substantial and compelling evidence that, in addition to its requirement for skeletal integrity, vitamin D sufficiency reduces the risk of development of a number of cancers, contributes to cardiovascular health, and stimulates immune response.

We also heard from Susan J. Whiting, Ph.D., Professor of Nutrition and Dietetics at the University of Saskatchewan, Saskatoon, Canada:

We know from intake studies that people cannot get much more than 200 IU per day. There's not enough choice in the marketplace nor [adequate] levels in existing foods. That means almost everyone needs a supplement. One must realize that risk/benefit is not confined to high doses. Not taking enough is a risk.

And from William B. Grant, Ph.D., of the Sunlight, Nutrition and Health Research Center (SUNARC) of San Francisco, California:

How could the IOM committee have set such low guidelines for vitamin D in light of the large body of evidence that vitamin D has important health benefits affecting risk of many types of disease? While the committee claimed it made a thorough review and assessment of over 1,000 studies and reports [Ross et al., 2010], they ignored 49,000 other papers on vitamin D listed at www.pubmed.gov.

Taken together, this evidence suggests that vitamin D plays a central role in regulating the expression of genes and proteins that prevent and inhibit cancer. The evidence of vitamin D's influence on key biological functions vital to health and well-being mandates that vitamin D no longer be ignored by our government, by the healthcare industry, or by individuals striving to achieve and maintain a greater state of health.

Can vitamin D play a role in treating cancer, not just its prevention? Yes. The cancer-stopping potential of vitamin D has been well-documented. Up to the point of massive differentiation, cancer cells maintain vitamin-D receptors that make them susceptible to the anticancer effects of this vitamin-hormone.

Vitamin D supplements and vitamin D–rich foods including salmon, tuna, and fish oils all contribute to transitioning the cancer cells from a near-term threat into a long-term manageable condition. If a cell has already undergone malignant transformation, activated vitamin D can team up with other proteins to stimulate programmed death of abnormal cells, the process known as cell apoptosis.

There's more good news. A growing body of evidence shows that a higher intake of vitamin D may be helpful in the prevention and treatment of high blood pressure, fibromyalgia, diabetes, multiple sclerosis, rheumatoid arthritis, and other diseases.

Critics of vitamin D point to the potential for overdosing resulting in toxic levels of the vitamin in the bloodstream. Symptoms of vitamin D toxicity include the onset of anorexia, disorientation, dehydration, fatigue, weight loss, weakness, and vomiting. One study demonstrated these effects when a single-dose of 500,000 IU of vitamin D_3 was injected into a patient. A half-million IU at once seems irrationally high and no doubt can result in toxicity. But numerous studies show levels of 10,000 IU per day to be safe. The fact is vitamin D toxicity is very rare.

As previously noted, the skin produces approximately 10,000 IU vitamin D in response to fifteen to twenty minutes summer sun exposure. However, most people do not receive fifteen to twenty minutes of sun exposure daily. This is especially true in northern and southern latitudes during their winter months. When well adults and adolescents are regularly deprived of adequate sunlight exposure, research indicates the advisability to supplement with at least 2,000 units (IU) of vitamin D daily.

It is important to supplement with vitamin D_3 rather than vitamin D_2, a synthetic form of the vitamin made by irradiating fungus and plant matter. D_2 is the form of vitamin D typically prescribed by doctors. This is not the type produced by your body in response to sun exposure. A recent meta-analysis by the Cochrane Database looked at fifty randomized controlled trials that included nearly 100,000 participants. The results showed a relative risk reduction among those who used vitamin D_3 but a relative risk increase among those who used D_2.

Further research shows vitamin D_3 is nearly 90 percent more potent in raising and maintaining vitamin D levels in the blood than D_2. It also produces vitamin D storage levels two to three times greater than D_2 and is converted into its active form much faster.

The critical factor is your serum level of vitamin D. Ideally this should be maintained between 50–70 ng/mL (nanograms per milliliter). I suggest you begin taking vitamin D_3 and, at your next doctor's appointment, ask for a blood test to determine your levels. Adjust your vitamin D supplementation based on those tests.

What does all this mean? It means you have a decision to make. But the facts are clear. We now have hundreds of studies to show that most North Americans who live above the 36th-degree parallel, a line that runs roughly from Los Angeles, California, through Atlanta, Georgia, are deficient in vitamin D. That deficiency has been correlated with a host of diseases, most notably breast and prostate cancers but also ovarian, pancreatic, and head and neck cancers.

I have been at this work for over a quarter century. In our early days, the science was not there to support our common-sense claims regarding nutrition and exercise in integrated cancer care. Today the scientific evidence is overwhelming, especially the evidence for vitamin D supplementation. But it is now ignored by our governments. This is exceedingly frustrating and totally unacceptable.

Decide for yourself. I stand firmly by our recommendations for healthy adults to supplement with vitamin D at the rate of 2,000 IU per day, 5,000 IU daily if you are dealing with a cancer diagnosis. See section #25 of this book, "Determine Your Nutritional Supplement Program" for further details.

This much I believe to be true: with vitamin D supplementation we can now prevent nearly 80 percent of all breast cancers and over 50 percent of all prostate cancers. This is actual prevention, not early detection or early intervention. It is also clear to me that vitamin D significantly helps in making cancer treatments more effective.

Those are huge promises. I believe vitamin D delivers. And I further believe vitamin D will revolutionize the way cancer is prevented and treated.

CANCER AND SUGAR

Q: Does sugar "feed" cancer cells?
A: Yes, indirectly.

Q: Can sugar cause other health conditions that can lead to cancer?
A: Definitely.

Q: Should I limit my sugar consumption?
A: Absolutely.

Contrary to popular belief, a calorie is not a calorie. Sugar certainly contains calories, "empty" calories. But sugar is also toxic and addictive.

Last month my wife and I attended a party hosted by a cancer charity. A breast cancer patient, Maria, just seven months postchemotherapy, was in attendance. I was enjoying a glass of red wine when Maria introduced herself. "No alcohol for me," she proclaimed. "You know how alcohol turns right into sugar and feeds those cancer cells."

I don't mind being held accountable for my dietary choices or the warnings about which I write. But when I looked at Maria's drink, I had to return her reminder. She was drinking coffee. "What's that?" I said, pointing to her cup. "Coffee," Maria replied. Noticing the light brown color I asked, "And what did you add to your coffee?" Maria blushed. "Cream—and sugar," she answered.

In the field of cancer research, there exists a subspecialty of inquiry with big potential—very big potential. It is called "cancer metabolism." This area of investigation combines cellular physiology and nutrition. It is an area long overdue for inquiry. To date, cancer metabolism's major contribution is to help us understand that cancer cells need more nutrition, more of a specific type of nutrient, in order to survive. This brings us directly to the issue of glucose, a cancer cell's preferred nutrient.

We have known about cancer metabolism for decades. In 1931, the Nobel Prize in medicine was awarded to Otto Warburg, M.D., Ph.D. This German genius was the first to discover that cancer cells have a fundamentally different metabolic process than healthy cells. Warburg posited that carcinogens are not the primary cause of cancer but are a secondary cause. He demonstrated that the prime cause of cancer is ". . . the replacement of oxygen in the respiratory chemistry of normal cells by (a fermentation of) sugar." Warburg's work produced a bio-physiological model that explained how too much glucose, sucrose, and fructose wreak havoc by starving normal cells of adequate oxygen supplies. The result: impaired immune function.

Warburg's work was widely criticized by many in the cancer industry as "too simplistic." But now, nearly eighty years later, interest in his discovery has resurfaced and new research in cancer metabolism and metabolic syndrome is finally being conducted. The key point to date: scientists can now demonstrate that controlling blood glucose levels within an optimal range actually bolsters immune function.

But controlling blood sugar levels is no easy task, especially if one favors the typical Western diet, which consists of lots of processed foods and meats, lots of added fats and hidden sweeteners, plus lots of highly refined grains and cereals—lots of everything except fresh vegetables, fresh fruits, and whole grains. We now have indisputable evidence that populations who consume this diet invariably suffer from higher rates of the aptly named Western diseases, especially obesity, type 2 diabetes, the full range of cardiovascular conditions, as well as the most common cancers— breast, prostate, and colorectal.

The scientific evidence is overwhelming. Today the debate in nutritional science is no longer about the links between the Western diet and a host of diseases. Now the discussion has turned to identifying the specific culprit nutrients in that diet that are responsible for specific diseases. Is it the saturated fat? Trans fats? Maybe it's the refined carbohydrates. What about the lack of fiber? Or not enough omega fatty acids. This is an important and fascinating discussion to some of us. But whatever the specific nutrient culprits, as people who need to eat, even the least aware among us know we have a Western diet problem.

After nearly three decades of journalistic research on the link between diet and cancer, I have come to believe that that the culprit nutrient in the Western diet is sugar—more accurately, the excessive consumption of sugar.

By "sugar" I am referring not only to the refined white granulated kind that we may spoon into our coffee or sprinkle on our breakfast cereal, I am also including high-fructose corn syrup, or "corn sugar" as the corn products industry would now prefer it to be called. For our discussion, this means that "sugar" will be defined as both sucrose—cane as well as beet, white or brown—and fructose. This is an important point of understanding because the fructose, especially high-fructose corn syrup, is today hidden in thousands of the processed foods you and I routinely place on our dinner table and enjoy at our favorite restaurants.

If we are to be informed consumers, we need to understand that sugar is everywhere in our food supply. If our food is boxed or bottled or canned, it very likely has sugar in it. And more than just empty calories, the evidence is overwhelming that overindulgence in such foods is very harmful to our health. In fact, I now believe sugar must be thought of just like tobacco and alcohol, something that is killing us—a man-made epidemic that requires a societal and governmental response.

Approximately thirty years ago, high-fructose corn syrup began to replace sugar in carbonated beverages. At that point in time, refined sugar was starting to be seen as a questionable nutrient. High-fructose corn syrup was marketed by the food industry as a healthier choice. Soon it began to appear in many prepared foods. But it wasn't a healthier choice.

For the more technical among us, refined sugar, also known as sucrose, consists of a molecule of the carbohydrate glucose and a molecule of the carbohydrate fructose. It's a fifty-fifty mix of the two. It's the molecule of fructose, which is nearly twice as sweet as the glucose, which distinguishes refined sugar from other car-

bohydrate-heavy foods like potatoes and bread that upon diges-
tion break down to glucose alone. The essential point is that the
more fructose in a substance, the sweeter it will be.

High-fructose corn syrup is sweeter than refined sugar. As it is
most commonly used in processed foods, it is approximately 55
percent fructose and 45 percent glucose. That extra fructose ends
up in our digestive tracks and directly impacts our blood sugar
levels and ultimately our immune function.

In 2009, Robert H. Lustig, M.D., UCSF Professor of Pediatrics
in the Division of Endocrinology, gave a lecture called "Sugar:
The Bitter Truth." It explored the damage caused by sugary
foods. He argues that fructose (too much) and fiber (not enough)
appear to be cornerstones of the obesity epidemic through their
effects on insulin. The video of that lecture is posted on YouTube
and has been viewed over 2.6 million times, an amazing number
of hits for a ninety-minute discussion on the biochemistry of
sugar.

In 2011, Gary Taubes wrote an article for the *New York Times
Magazine* entitled "Is Sugar Toxic?" A good deal of the article ana-
lyzes the Lustig's lecture. Taubes writes:

> If Lustig is right, then our excessive consumption of sugar is
> the primary reason that the numbers of obese and diabetic
> Americans have skyrocketed in the past 30 years. But his
> argument implies more than that . . . it would mean that
> sugar is also the likely dietary cause of several other chronic
> ailments widely considered to be diseases of Western life-
> styles—heart disease, hypertension and many common
> cancers.

Even the underinformed among us know the empty calories
argument against sugar.

But Lustig and Taubes go far beyond the empty calories warnings. They both help us understand that the human body me-
tabolizes sugar, specifically the fructose in sugar, in a way that
makes it toxic and harmful when consumed in large quantities.

The main difference: glucose is processed by all cells in our body. But the fructose in sugar and in high-fructose corn syrup is processed by our liver, one of the critical organs in immune function. Herein lies the problem and the direct connection with cancer.

The Corn Refiners Association's Website, SweetSurprise.com, states ". . . research confirms that high fructose corn syrup is safe and no different from other common sweeteners like table sugar and honey. All three sweeteners are nutritionally the same." The site goes on to proclaim that ". . . though individual sugars are metabolized by different pathways, this is of little consequence since the body sees the same mix of sugars from caloric sweeteners, regardless of source."

I beg to differ. In a study published in 2005 in the journal *Cancer Research*, the authors noted that the way different sugars are processed using different metabolic pathways is of "major" consequence in cancer. This study found that cancer cells readily metabolize fructose to increase their proliferation. In this case they were studying pancreatic cancer, one of the most deadly forms of cancer. The research documented the unique role of fructose in cell division and the resulting growth and spread of the disease.

We know beyond doubt from decades of laboratory studies that when fructose arrives at the liver in sufficient quantities, much of it will be converted to fat. This produces what is called insulin resistance and which in turn is now understood as one of the fundamental causes of obesity. Of course insulin resistance is also implicated in diabetes, heart disease, and now many types of cancers. Fat accumulation in the liver as a result of the excessive consumption of sugar is the key point to understand. The essential finding is that our ability to metabolize the high quantities of hidden fructose is compromised and the result is insulin resistance. Interestingly, this is absolutely parallel with Otto Warburg's discovery and understanding of nearly eighty years ago.

We also know from the World Health Organization's extensive nutritional research efforts that there is a demonstrated link between obesity, diabetes, and cancer. Simply put, if you are obese and diabetic you are statistically more likely to be diagnosed with cancer than someone who is not. This finding is virtually parallel with the previous observations on the sugar-rich Western diet. The problem is so significant that even age-adjusted death rates from cancer are rising in North America. For example, this means that the likelihood of any one fifty-five-year-old female dying from breast cancer is increasing, even as there are more fifty-five-year-old females.

What is the physiological mechanism that leads from insulin resistance to a diagnosis of cancer? Many endocrinologists now believe that once insulin resistance sets in, this signals our pancreas to secrete more insulin. And insulin, as well as a related hormone called insulin-like growth factor, actually promotes tumor growth. The evidence is mounting that many pre-cancerous cells would not become malignant unless they were signaled by insulin to take up more blood sugar. This physiology is the essential root of the old adage "sugar feeds cancer." And after four decades of debate, the old adage seems to be proving true.

There's more on sugar and cancer. I will simplify the scientifically validated information:

- There is definitive proof that when malignant tumors process sugar they create lactic acid. Two things happen in the process:
  - First, the lactic acid is transported to the liver and as a result generates a more acidic pH level. Lactic acid likely drives the extreme fatigue that is so common in cancer patients.
  - Second, the combination of the lactic acid and fat accumulation in the liver makes for inefficient energy metabolism. This means cancer patients are often able to extract just a small percentage of nutrient value from their food. This leads to malnutrition and the "wasting" condition so many cancer patients experience.
- There is one other extensively researched sugar-cancer connection. This relates to simple carbohydrates and how they

are processed by our bodies. Refined flour, used in the making of bread, is a perfect example. "White" bread is broken down by the digestive process into sugar—glucose and sucrose. Not only do these sugars increase the burden on the liver, excellent scientific evidence shows they also decrease the ability of white blood cells, specifically the type called neutrophils, to help destroy invaders such as precancerous cells.

It all adds up to a vicious cycle. It leads me to conclude that all forms of sugar are detrimental to health. Even more, because of the deleterious effects on liver function, all sugars promote cancer, albeit in slightly different ways and to a different extent. But most important, fructose is clearly the most harmful.

Please recognize the connection: sugar—decreased liver function—decreased immune function—increased risk of cancer.

What does this mean? As for me, I will not consume sugar, especially high-fructose corn syrup, if I can possibly avoid it. I believe absolutely minimizing sugar is something we can all do to significantly decrease our risk of developing cancer and to greatly increase our odds of survival. I am urging you to do the same.

Contrary to standard advice from the oncology community, you should not eat whatever you want. Wise nutritional choices are critically important to cancer prevention and survival. Believe it, diet very much matters—especially your intake of sugar. Minimize sugar.

CLEAN OUT YOUR PANTRY AND REFRIGERATOR

Your refrigerator and pantry are likely to contain processed foods. If ever there was a time to eat real food, cancer is it. Now I ask you to take a bold step toward making thoughtful choices about nutrition.

1. Throw out the following oils:

a. Margarine
b. Solid shortenings
c. Partially hydrogenated oil
. . . or products made with them

2. Buy the following oils:

a. Extra virgin olive oil
b. Vegetable spray
c. Sesame oil

3. Throw out the following sweeteners:

a. Sugar
b. Aspartame
c. Saccharin
. . . or products made with them

4. Buy the following sweetener:

a. Stevia

5. Throw out the following meats:

a. Salami
b. Bologna
c. Sausage
d. Bacon
e. Hot dogs
f. Smoked ham
g. Smoked turkey
. . . or products made with them

Once you clean out the shelves, you're on your way to bringing health to your dinner plate.

Cook and Shop Healthfully

Healthy Cooking Techniques:

1. Coat the pan with vegetable spray
2. Stir-fry
3. Oven-fry
4. Bake in parchment or foil
5. Poach
6. Steam
7. Stew

SEASON HEALTHFULLY USING HERBS AND SPICES

To Flavor:	Use:
Vegetables	Basil, caraway, chives, dill, ginger, tarragon, oregano, rosemary
Fruits	Cinnamon, cloves, mint, nutmeg
Meats	Garlic, oregano, rosemary, sage, dill, fennel, tarragon, thyme, parsley, curry powder
Salads	Basil, chives, dill, marjoram, mint, parsley

Shop Healthfully

1. Read labels.
2. Buy lowest fat/salt/sugar choices.
3. Eat before you shop.

SAMPLE MENUS

Countless times I have been asked for sample meal plans. I am pleased to offer here two variations with two options for each meal. With simple substitutions, you can create a joyful variety of delicious meals that maximize nutrition.

The Cancer Recovery Foundation Meal Plan: "Three Squares" a Day

MEAL #1

Option A:

Scrambled egg whites with red peppers and onions
Tomato slices
Orange
Herb tea

Option B:

Oatmeal

Soy milk
Blueberries
Ginger tea

MEAL #2

Option A:

Chicken Caesar salad with whole grain croutons
Carrot sticks with hummus
Iced green tea

Option B:

Veggie burger with whole grain bread
Mixed green salad
Fresh tomato juice

MEAL #3

Option A:

Baked eggplant
Whole grain dinner roll
Steamed broccoli
Mixed green salad
Apple slices

Option B:

Wild salmon
Brown rice
Mashed cauliflower
Greek salad
Fresh plum

The Cancer Recovery Foundation Meal Plan:
Six "Mini-Meals" a Day

MEAL #1

Option A:

Fresh tomato juice
Whole wheat bagel/peanut butter

Option B:

Grapefruit
Hard-boiled egg

MEAL #2

Option A:

Mixed green salad

Option B:

Non-fat yogurt

MEAL #3

Option A:

Vegetable soup
Cheese

Option B:

Mixed green salad
Almonds

MEAL #4

Option A:

Protein bar (sugar-free)

Option B:

Apple

MEAL #5

Option A:

Herb-encrusted fish
Mixed green salad

Option B:

Roast turkey breast
Mashed cauliflower

MEAL #6

Option A:

Non-fat Greek yogurt

Option B:

Celery sticks with hummus

The Cancer Recovery "Real Foods" Shopping List™

Vegetable
____Broccoli
____Cabbage
____Peppers
____Tomatoes
____Carrots
____Leaf lettuce
____Cauliflower
____Onions
____Beets
____Asparagus
____Squash
____Pumpkin

Fish and Meat
____Cod/flounder
____Tilapia
____Salmon (wild)
____Tuna
____Trout
____Mahi-mahi
____Sardines
____Haddock
____Skinless chicken breast
____Skinless turkey breast

Legumes
____Black beans
____Garbanzo beans
____Kidney beans
____Navy beans
____Pinto beans
____Lentils
____Split peas

Non-fat Dairy
____Yogurt
____Cottage cheese
____Almond milk

Fruit
____Berries
____Oranges
____Red grapefruit
____Mangoes
____Apples
____Cherries
____Apricots
____Cantaloupe
____Kiwis
____Pears
____Red grapes
____Watermelon

Whole Grains and Breads
____Oats and oatmeal
____Barley
____Brown rice
____Flaxseed
____Buckwheat
____Spelt wheat
____Millet
____Amaranth
____Quinoa
____Wheat germ

Other
____Garlic
____Ginger
____Cinnamon
____Cayenne
____Stevia
____Green tea
____Curry powder

Oils
____Extra virgin olive oil
____Sesame oil
____Non-fat vegetable spray

Feel free to copy this list and bring it with you to the market.

GUIDE 2:
MIND/BODY
AND HEALING

ILLNESS REPRESENTATIONS

The Mind/Body Connection Matures

My wife and I began our work in 1985, just months after I was told by my surgeon, "I'd give you about thirty days to live." At that time a book called *Love, Medicine and Miracles* by Bernie Siegel, M.D., was just making its debut. The book's release was widely embraced by the media. Soon I found a copy and began to devour it.

Dr. Siegel's experience as a surgeon led him to become aware that those patients, especially cancer patients, who held expectations of a positive outcome often did better than those patients who simply gave up. This led him and his wife, Bobbi, to form a group he called ECaP (Exceptional Cancer Patients). They held support group meetings, and central to the experience was the practice of mind/body techniques. Many different meditative disciplines were taught at ECaP, as well as the concept that mind and body worked together to positively impact health. "Bernie," as he preferred to be called, through his books and public appearances, did much to popularize the mind/body movement as it applied to cancer and healing.

Others came before Bernie, including Herbert Benson, M.D., and Lawrence LeShan, Ph.D. Both made significant and lasting contributions to our understanding of the mind/body connection. But the foremost pioneer in modern-day psychosocial oncology was O. Carl Simonton, M.D. (1942–2009). Trained as a physician at the University of Oregon Medical School, Simonton completed a three-year residency in radiation oncology. It was during this time that he developed a model of emotional support for the treatment of cancer patients. As Chief of Radiation Oncology at Travis Air Force Base, Simonton first implemented the model. Dr. Simonton's work was the first systematic emotional intervention used in the treatment of cancer. His program was actually approved by the Surgeon General's Office in 1973. Simonton was the pioneer who introduced and applied the concept that one's state of mind could influence one's ability to survive cancer.

This idea was revolutionary. Enthusiastically received by cancer patients, Simonton's work was widely condemned by the medical community. Oncologists derided the idea that the mind and emotions had a role in either the onset of cancer or in the recovery from it. The American Cancer Society put Simonton's model on their so-called blacklist of dangerous unproven methods, an unfortunate derogatory characterization that would remain with Simonton through the 1990s.

The groundbreaking Simonton Cancer Program was founded on ten major tenets. Dr. Simonton postulated:

1. Our emotions significantly influence health and recovery from disease (including cancer). Emotions are a strong driving force in the immune system and other healing systems.
2. Our beliefs and attitudes influence our emotions, thereby affecting our health and healing systems.
3. We can significantly influence our beliefs and attitudes.

As a result, we shape our emotions, and therefore, significantly influence our health.

4. Ways of influencing beliefs, attitudes and emotions can be readily taught and learned by using a variety of accessible methods that are presented in this (Simonton) program.

5. All of us function as physical, mental, social and spiritual/philosophical beings. These aspects need to be addressed in the broad context of healing, with a focus on the particular needs of a person who is ill, and that person's family, community, and culture.

6. Harmony is central to health—balance among the physical, mental, and spiritual/philosophical aspects of being. This extends to relationships with self, family, friends, community, planet, and universe.

7. We have inherent (genetic, instinctual) tendencies and abilities that aid us in moving in the direction of health and harmony (physical, mental, spiritual/philosophical and social).

8. These abilities can be developed and implemented in meaningful ways through existing techniques and methods that are presented in this program.

9. As these abilities are developed, proficiency evolves, as when learning other skills. The result is greater harmony and improved quality of life, which significantly impacts one's state of health.

10. These skills and insights also change our relationship with death by lessening our fear and pain, and freeing more energy for getting well and living life more fully today.

A New Era in Mind/Body Approaches

Many pioneering medical efforts prove to be less than complete, even dangerous. Not so with Simonton's. His work has stood the test and is now being confirmed in the new and burgeoning field of health psychology called illness representations. These new insights and understandings are creating a revolution in mind/body medicine.

Illness representations are a patient's beliefs and expectations about a symptom or illness and how those beliefs and expectations actually impact the experience and outcome of the symptom or illness. An example may best explain this construct.

Assume a healthy person starts to feel slightly achy and begins to experience a runny nose. The individual identifies and then "labels" the symptoms as most likely the beginning of the common cold. Since this person believes a cold to be a temporary phenomenon lasting perhaps a week to ten days, a "timeline" is now added to the initial label. And the initial label of a common cold instills a belief that the symptoms, and any resulting illness, present a minor threat. Thus the "consequences" of a cold are not believed to be serious.

This individual may also think, *I know where I got this. Harry at work was sneezing and coughing for a couple of days. That's it.* Thus a "cause" is assigned. This leads to the individual's beliefs about colds and how they are best managed. *Okay*, he thinks. *I need to drink lots of fluids, get extra rest, and have chicken soup a couple of times a day.* This reflects the individual's beliefs about a "cure" for the common cold.

There are parallel emotional reactions to each of these cognitive processes. And even though in the case of the common cold the emotions will tend to be subtle or muted, the emotions are nonetheless present. For many people the emotional reaction to a cold will be annoyance, *Oh no, I'll probably have to miss work and this will put an extra burden on my coworkers to meet the project deadline.* Or the emotional impact could be concern about the cold being a precursor to a more serious health problem. The emotional response to the individual's beliefs is called "illness coherence."

Cancer typically triggers a completely different set of beliefs and emotional responses. As an illustration, let's assume a woman detects an unusual lump in her breast. For millions of women, the first thought (label) that comes to mind is breast cancer. This suspicious-lump-equals-breast-cancer belief runs deep and often sets in motion a complex combination of personal and cultural beliefs. The cluster of thoughts that tend to be fused together with very intense emotions include *breast cancer runs in my family* (cause), *this is going to mean surgery and the dreaded chemotherapy* (cure), *breast cancer is serious, even life-threatening* (consequences), *this will mean a year or two of treatment and uncertainty* (timeline), *and I may die* (illness coherence). It's easy to see why cancer is called a "hot cognition."

Several researchers are now dedicated to understanding illness representations more fully. But the pioneer is clearly Howard Leventhal, Ph.D., Director of the Rutgers Center for the Study of Health Beliefs and Behaviors, Institute of Health, Department of Psychology at Rutgers University in New Jersey. Leventhal and his colleagues have broken new ground in the understanding of the mind's role in health and healing. And consistent with Simonton, the central point of understanding is that our emotions greatly impact our health and prospects for recovery from illness.

One of the Leventhal team's most basic discoveries is that patients are only partially aware of how they create and maintain personal views of disease and treatment. And in the case of cancer, the typical beliefs are detrimental to recovery, healing, and maintenance of health.

In our work we have found the belief that cancer equates with death to be very widely held. Countless times I have listened as patients maintain their views and defend their beliefs, even if those beliefs are harmful. For tens of thousands of cancer patients, the mind-set is, "Yes, I will fight. I'll do anything to survive. But in the end, my cancer is probably going to kill me."

About three years ago, a gentleman going through prostate cancer was in my office. His surgery followed by hormone therapy was successful in controlling the cancer. And even though he suffered from incontinence and impotence following treatment, his follow-up tests showed no signs of cancer. In an effort to instill a more upward look, I proclaimed, "Celebrate with me, Omar. You are a survivor!" His answer foreshadowed a different outcome. He said, "You know, Greg, I'm doing well now, but this kind of cancer always gets you." We examined his belief, but to limited avail. I spoke at his funeral service about four years following his initial diagnosis.

As stated in the "50 Essential Things to Do" section on beliefs, cancer absolutely does not equate with death. This is a very harmful toxic illness representation. For patients who want to get well and stay well, illness representations that equate cancer and death must be changed.

Simonton was one of the first to ask patients to illustrate their cancer and their treatment. He gave them a small box of crayons and one sheet of paper and said, "Draw your cancer and your treatment." The objective was to help the patient gain a greater understanding of the beliefs they brought to the recovery process. For example, a person who illustrated their illness as a mountainous rock formation and their treatment as a mere hand shovel were led to explore the beliefs behind those images. In the end, one hoped the power of the images of treatment would match the power of the images of the illness. We continue to implement variations of this exercise in our work today.

Traditional mind/body techniques have their place. Transcendental Meditation, and is less-religious offspring the relaxation response, can clearly help counter stress. They also assist in lowering blood pressure and changing other vital bodily functions that are normally unconscious. Biofeedback and mindfulness meditation yield similar results. But none demonstrate the physiological outcomes like illness representations—the new frontier in mind/body understanding.

The Power of Awareness

There is a great deal to be gained when cancer patients better understand the way in which they are processing their experience. We are now aware that illness representations have a predictive validity that can significantly assist patients in examining their beliefs and attitudes toward a cancer diagnosis.

New tools to assess illness representation are being developed around the globe. I would like to add to these efforts. I wish to acknowledge the work of Dr. Elizabeth Broadbent at the University of Auckland's School of Medicine for allowing me to borrow from her work in developing this tool specifically for cancer patients.

THE CANCER REPRESENTATION QUESTIONNAIRE (SHORT FORM)

FOR THE FOLLOWING QUESTIONS, PLEASE CIRCLE THE NUMBER THAT BEST CORRESPONDS TO YOUR VIEW.

1. Once your symptoms were diagnosed (labeled) as "cancer," how much impact has the diagnosis had on your life?

   0   1   2   3   4   5   6   7   8   9   10

   Severe   No
   impact   impact

2. How long do you think your cancer will be active (timeline)?

   0   1   2   3   4   5   6   7   8   9   10

   As long   A very
   as I live   short time

3. How much personal control do you feel you have over your illness (control)?

   0   1   2   3   4   5   6   7   8   9   10

   Absolutely   Significant
   no control   control

4. How much do you think your treatment can help your illness (cure)?

   0   1   2   3   4   5   6   7   8   9   10

   Not at all   Very helpful

5. How much do you experience symptoms from your illness (consequences)?

   0   1   2   3   4   5   6   7   8   9   10

   Many severe   No symptoms
   symptoms   at all

6. How much do you experience symptoms from your cancer treatment (consequences)?

   0   1   2   3   4   5   6   7   8   9   10

   Many severe   No symptoms
   symptoms   at all

7. How concerned are you about your illness (consequences)?

   0   1   2   3   4   5   6   7   8   9   10

   Extremely   No concern
   concerned   at all

8. How well do you understand the clinical aspects of you diagnosis (control)?

   0   1   2   3   4   5   6   7   8   9   10

   Do not   Very clear
   understand   understanding

9. How much does your diagnosis and treatment affect you emotionally? For example, does it make you angry, depressed, frightened, or upset (coherence)?

   0   1   2   3   4   5   6   7   8   9   10

   Extremely emotionally   No emotional
   impacted   change

10. How much do you believe you personally contributed to your cancer diagnosis (cause)?

0   1   2   3   4   5   6   7   8   9   10

Absolutely   I greatly
no contribution   contributed

Please total your scores from questions 1 through 10. Record
total here_____
Please list in order of priority the three most important factors
that you believe caused your illness:

A. _____
B. _____
C. _____

The interpretation and predictive value of illness perceptions and responses are as much art as science. But generally,
either a low score (0–15) or a high score (85–100) indicate extreme responses to a cancer diagnosis. Neither is preferred.
Midrange scores indicate a balanced response, which is
preferred.

The scores are indicative of the "intensity of beliefs" regarding a cancer diagnosis and subsequent treatment. But it is
neither the score nor the beliefs that matter. It is the emotions
generated by the beliefs and simply indicated by the score.
The good news is that we can change our beliefs and thus our
emotions. Awareness of our beliefs is the starting point.

Is the Glass Half Full or Half Empty?

The subject of illness representation quickly leads to the question of positive thinking—a state of mind that is deeply imbed-
ded in the beliefs we hold. Over the past quarter-century, my
work has been the leading voice of the positive thinking school in
the cancer field. Through our work we have encouraged literally
millions of cancer patients to change their negative beliefs into
positive expectations. Unapologetically, I want people to embrace hope and the possibility for healing.

This message is not universally appealing. Many patients have made it clear that in their eyes I am naïve, uninformed, and even cruel. "Positive thinking? Is that all it takes to cure my lung cancer?" wrote a patient. "You've got to be kidding. Are you sure you had lung cancer?" Another e-mailed, "You can talk about hope all day long. But there are days I just need to cry."

Jerome Groopman, M.D., is an oncologist and author of the book *The Anatomy of Hope*. The book chronicles patients who he considers were helped by positive hopeful thinking and some whose demise he attributes, in large part, to lack of hope. Groopman's studies show that positive beliefs and expectations—the essential contents of hope—impact the body on a physiological level. Pain management, respiration, circulation, and even motor function are demonstrated to be enhanced with a positive outlook.

I have never represented the view that all it takes to cure cancer is positive thinking. But I have long advocated that a person with cancer is best served by beliefs and attitudes that project an upward look. Evidence has existed for decades that immunoglobulin levels, a precursor and one measurement of immune function, increase with a more hopeful stance. Yet as soon as I put forward this evidence and make the positive outlook assertion, there is a small but vocal group of patients who respond, "Stop laying a guilt trip on me. You're saying, at some level, I caused my cancer." Not so.

The hopeful outlook bolsters health—emotionally and physically. It produces a sense of guilt only if that is how it is received. Today we can note the further evidence from the field of illness representation leads to a profound conclusion: belief and hope are very real and very powerful forces in health and healing. And there is a biology connected to positive thinking.

Of course this is interpreted as "false hope" by many people. But once again, I firmly believe there is no such thing as false hope. I believe there is only real hope—for a cure, for a peaceful death, for a better tomorrow no matter how long we may have to live.

Unfortunately, there is a very real and toxic force called "false no-hope." This is typically when the doctor finds it necessary to give patients the "get your affairs in order" speech. It is a devastating experience. I can still clearly recall how despondent I became after my surgeon gave me thirty days to live. Every week we counsel frightened and depressed patients who have been given a terminal diagnosis.

Our guidance to these patients has changed over the decades. I used to encourage everyone who received the "terminal" news to actively and forcefully challenge the doctor. My advice was helpful to only a few and probably created what some called a positive thinking prison for some patients.

Today we encourage cancer patients to experience all their feelings and help them understand that fear and despair are normal natural responses to a life-threatening illness. Face it, some days following chemotherapy are lousy. The bone-deep fatigue that often comes with radiation therapy generates understandable thoughts of hopelessness. One patient remarked, "If I started to feel bad, I began to think there was something wrong with me."

Now we teach, "Feel the feelings—the positive as well as the negative. But do not get into the habit of replaying the negatives ones." Repeatedly rehearsing our ills is a trap even more deadly than denial. We remind patients that all our emotions are rooted in our beliefs—and beliefs are things we have the absolute power to change.

Positive thinking? Yes. Optimism? Of course. As long as they lead to feelings of hope. Positive thinking and optimism are cognitive behaviors—decisions. Hope is an emotion, a feeling that differentiates this force from merely choosing an upward look.

Our emotions make the difference. And it is the hopeful emotional response that serves us best in our illness representations.

Welcome to the new era of mind/body medicine.

MEDITATION AND VISUALIZATION EXERCISES

You may decide to choose a mind/body exercise to integrate into your healing program. There is excellent evidence that many mind/body/spirit approaches can play an important role in the healing process.

Meditation produces demonstrable effects on brain and immune function. Some of the side effects of conventional cancer treatments may be lessened with the integration of simple meditative exercises. Meditation includes a wide range of approaches. The exercises described below are those that have been helpful to thousands of cancer patients around the world.

Meditation

For many of us, our minds are so busy with thoughts that we rarely create the opportunity to simply be at peace, relaxing into the present moment, quieting our minds, and being more aware of the sensations in our bodies.

By practicing meditation, which is simply learning to relax and be at peace, we can become more open and attentive to our deeper, intuitive wisdom and the healing potential that lies within us. By invoking this relaxation response, our body moves into the parasympathetic "healing" mode in which physical healing is optimized.

Meditation is a way of cultivating moment-to-moment awareness and supports becoming more present to our own experience. To do this requires that we become aware of the constant stream of thoughts and reactions to our inner and outer experiences in which we are all normally caught up. During meditation or contemplation, we discover that we are constantly generating thoughts and reactions. By simply becoming aware of our breath instead of the stream of thoughts, we become more aware of our body experience, allowing us to release pent-up anxieties and emotions. With practice we can move toward acceptance and release of stress, and even change our limiting beliefs.

Meditation is a valuable way of reestablishing inner calmness and balance in the face of emotional upset or when you "have a lot on your mind." When life becomes stressful and out of balance, we have all experienced how relaxing it can be to be alone for a few minutes and just breathe, in and out, deeply and quietly. Research has shown that meditation can alleviate psychological and physical suffering of persons living with cancer.

Visualization

Guided imagery, also known as visualization, is an extension of meditation. A leader or a recorded script is often employed to assist the participant in visualizing health and healing. Guided imagery has been credited with reducing side effects, pain, and stress. It can also aid in emotional coping with cancer and assist in preparing for anticipated situations such as surgery or chemotherapy. The imagery process can also be helpful in decision-making and can be employed to improve mental health and control. Finally, guided imagery can reduce the need for pain medication. Research shows increases in natural killer cell activity as a result.

Both meditation and guided imagery are less about method and more about calming your mind and spirit and living in the present moment. By cultivating clarity and peace in meditation, by imaging health and healing, we become more accepting, less judgmental, and happier. What follows are some suggested scripts for your consideration:

Meditation Exercise: Relaxation

Please try this simple exercise to help you fully relax your body:

- Close your eyes, remove glasses, loosen tight clothing, and take your shoes off.
- Start by adjusting your position so that you are sitting comfortably. Don't cross your legs, ankles or feet, or hands. Sit with your back supported. If your legs are too short to reach the floor comfortably, then put a book or bag on the floor on which to rest your feet. Lie on the floor if you wish.

- There may be sounds in the room or outside. Try to ignore them. Remember that life goes on and that we can become relaxed despite the noises around us.
- Raise your shoulders up to your ears and let them fall down gently.
- Open your mouth as if yawning, close it a little, and rock your lower jaw left and right.
- Close your mouth and push your tongue hard up to the roof of your mouth. Let the tongue spring back. Loosen your jaw more.
- Once again raise your shoulders to your ears, then release them gently.
- Now just breathe normally and softly.
- Allow your inward breath to become a little deeper.
- As you breathe, just notice the breath and bring your attention to the sensation of the breath flowing at the tip of your nostrils.
- Now notice the natural gentle movement of your chest as you breathe in and breathe out.
- Take a deep breath without straining.
- Allow the breath to come and go effortlessly.
- Just continue for a moment or two longer.
- Allow the natural rise and fall of your breath to help you to soften and relax and remove any tiredness or tension.
- As you breathe in, bring in softness and relaxation.
- As you exhale, take away any tiredness or tension.
- Inward breath bringing softness and relaxation.
- Outward breath taking away tension.
- Continue to breathe slowly and peacefully.
- Check around your body. Is there any remaining tension or tiredness? If so, take your breath there to soften and renew.

Visualization Exercise:
Guided Imagery for Healing

Please try this simple exercise to help you support immune function:

- Find a comfortable place to sit, with your back straight and your feet firmly on the ground. Ensure that you will not be disturbed during your meditation by muting your cell phone or taking your phone off the hook and allowing the answering machine to handle incoming calls.
- Take about five minutes to relax your body completely, working through from the feet up to the head. Imagine that you can just let go of all the muscles; feel them soften and release, allowing the tension to flow out of your whole being.
- Focus particularly on the shoulders, the neck, and the jaw, as these are areas where we often, without realizing it, hold a great deal of tension.
- When your body feels totally relaxed, bring your attention to your breathing. Don't change it. Just be aware of the breath moving in and out of your body.
- Notice as much as you can about your breathing. How it feels as the breath moves in and out of the nostrils? Where do you take the breath to in your body? Stay with this for another five minutes or so.
- Now imagine that you are outside in the sunshine. Get a sense of the light of the sun, warm but not too hot, and shining down on you. You might like to imagine that you are lying on a quiet beach soaking up the sunlight.
- Imagine that you can breathe in the light of the sun, taking it into your body. Let the light fill up every cell of your body. When you feel glowing and full of light, let that light move anywhere in your body where you feel that you are in need of healing. Feel your cells transforming, becoming energized as the radiance heals and restores you.
- Now let the light expand out of you. Radiate the light around

your body, so that you are imagining yourself glowing with light and health. Stay with this part of the meditation for about ten minutes.

- Now bring your attention back to the breath. Every time you breathe in, silently say, "I am breathing in health." And on each out-breath say to yourself, "I am happy and whole." As you do this, feel the truth of what you are saying. Believe it so that it becomes a reality for you.
- Now let it all go and bring yourself back to the room, slowly and gently. Feel the ground beneath your feet and become aware once more of your surroundings.

You may wish to expand your meditation and visualization experiences. Many communities offer classes that can assist you in perfecting these skills. There are also many recorded meditations that can be helpful in assisting your efforts.

GUIDE 3:
COMPLEMENTARY
CANCER THERAPIES

Two out of three cancer patients embrace one or more complementary or alternative practices. The information that follows is an overview of the major options. Your goal should be to obtain more complete information of the subjects that are of interest to you. Then you can design an appropriate integrated-care program of your own.

Question: When the subject is nontraditional cancer treatments, what should you expect from your oncologist?
Answer: Indifference.

For the most part, twenty-first-century oncology has limited time for, or interest in, complementary and alternative therapies. The biomedical model is tightly focused on surgery, radiation, chemotherapy, and hormonal therapy. Do not expect enthusiastic endorsements of approaches outside these core orthodox treatments.

If you were to expect anything beyond indifference, expect

criticism. The conventional cancer community's "party line" on diet, nutritional supplements, and other more natural treatment approaches remains decidedly negative. Only the rare oncologist will bridge the world between mainstream and complementary medicine, support you in the process of taking charge of your situation, and work step-by-step with you toward the recovery of your health.

Know this: a patient's interest in nontraditional cancer treatments is seen as a personal affront by most Western oncologists. It's as if the patient is saying, "Your ideas are not enough." Truth is, they are not. Do not expect to receive positive support for your complementary and alternative efforts from a conventionally trained and practicing oncologist.

You can typically expect more advice and support on complementary and self-help techniques from an informed nursing staff. The control of treatment side effects is the most common nurse-provided information. Their coaching might be expected to include both pharmaceutical options as well as more natural approaches. Look for referrals to community-based organizations for visualization, massage, relaxation, breathing techniques, comfort, and support.

Let's briefly review the most common components of integrated cancer care:

COUNSELING

Counseling within a holistic model is considered a central component of the healing process. Support through talking, through genuine give-and-take communication, is critical. It will help you become aware of your needs, define your questions, and determine how to go about receiving answers. In a real sense, this increased awareness is the heart of the entire holistic approach.

Millions carry a bias against counseling, thinking it is simply about relief of emotional distress. But transpersonal counseling, assisting to help the individual explore his or her needs from a whole-person perspective, is much more. Cancer challenges everything—from our physical body to our thoughts, feelings, significant relationships, and spirituality, as well as the environment in which we live.

While the initial focus of such counseling may be to help cope with the diagnosis and treatment of an individual's cancer, the counseling quickly becomes more expansive and even a cocreative experience. Discovery of the true self is both enlightening and supportive, encouraging the individual to access all resources—physical, emotional, and spiritual.

Perhaps the key issue of a transpersonal counseling approach is spiritual. It can help us identify what our soul and spirit are yearning for. Not surprisingly, a good number of cancer patients find ambiguity—on the surface they are engaged in actively fighting illness but at a deeper level they are blocked by a seemingly unsolvable problem that leads to despair or even the need to let go and die. Connecting with our deepest reality through transpersonal counseling often establishes great truth, peace and, ultimately, a healing of a higher order.

GROUP SUPPORT

Cancer Recovery Foundation's earliest work was focused exclusively on establishing psychospiritual support groups. The distinct advantage of this focus over a medical/clinical information approach is helping cancer patients discover the many abilities they possess and then implement them to overcome their present challenges. By focusing on what is possible, the aim is to give the individual a clear picture of the most effective way forward. Doing so within the context of mutual support among people in similar situations is extremely helpful.

The aim of group support is not to expose an individual's feelings. However, the process of group interaction can make it easier and safer for many people to express emotions, even safer than with family, friends, or a one-to-one counseling session. The group is also extremely effective in working together to identify common beliefs and patterns that may be obstructing progress towards self-acceptance and well-being.

CREATIVE THERAPIES

Art and music can bring freedom, giving people permission to express what they find difficult to put into words. These techniques require no previous training or even talent and ability. Often they are linked with group support. The central benefit is to release the more playful, joyful, and creative aspects of our individual natures. There is healing in the energy and fun we took for granted in our youth.

Art Therapy

Art therapy reconnects people with their own creativity. Work done in art therapy can help people discover a sense of empowerment and control in the often disempowering and out-of-control cancer experience. Art therapy can also be cathartic, releasing insights into recovery.

Creating with watercolors, acrylics, oils, charcoal, pens, markers, clay, paper, glue, or whatever they choose often suspends people in the moment, allowing them to become absorbed and involved. This is exceedingly beneficial in its own right because the mind can be at ease from its typical worries.

All art therapy is deemed to have high artistic merit. The symbols are important. It's joy and peace that the patient-artist is after. Positive expectations can be strengthened, emotional conflicts can be resolved, and a deepening awareness of one's spiritual dimension can be revealed—all through art therapy.

Music Therapy

Music has a long historical link with healing. The idea of music as a healing influence that could affect health and behavior is as least as old as the writings of Aristotle and Plato. Today a substantial body of research supports the efficacy of music therapy.

There are some common misconceptions about music therapy. That the patient has to have some particular music ability to benefit from music therapy—he or she does not. That there is one particular style of music that is more therapeutic than all the rest—this is not the case. All styles of music can be useful in effecting change in a patient's life. The individual's preferences, circumstances, and need for treatment, and the patient's goals help to determine the types of music he or she may use.

Be it actively playing music or simply listening to music, it has been demonstrated that music therapy can help people control anxiety, express feelings, lift spirits to a higher level, and even relieve pain. The positive shifts can result in a physiological boost.

SPIRITUAL HEALING

Spiritual healing, and for our purposes this will include laying on of hands, is perhaps the very oldest of the healing arts. This practice is part of the beliefs and practices of many religions. Based in the belief that we are all children of God, the practice seeks to reconnect the individual to the source that heals.

Increased connection with God certainly helps with coping. It can also dramatically improve one's understanding and acceptance of life circumstances. For many individuals, this reconnection further provides a strong reason for living, even a mission for one's life.

Spiritual healing can be brought about by prayer being offered by a healer or healers, by personal prayer, or by self-healing exercises. Spiritual healing rests in the belief that an individual's spirit, this universal life force that animates each of us, often becomes depleted. Through prayerful focused intention, the healer is able to tune in to that loving energy and bring it to whoever needs it, including themselves. The result is a restoration in the balance of body, mind, and spirit.

For the past two decades, I have studied with some of the most-respected and best-known healers. These various practitioners each have their own beliefs and practices. Results vary. However, there is this important insight: spiritual healing has its most powerful results when patients have their own strong personal beliefs and connect with a healer who shares those beliefs.

Lasting spiritual healing takes place in the quiet of one's spirit. For the most part, it will not be found in the arenas, on the stages, or under the television lights. There may be a celebration of healing in that environment, but the actual healing is found elsewhere.

I have repeatedly observed one important dynamic of spiritual healing. The turning point is to be found where the individual seeking healing expresses a sincere desire for, and an invitation asking for, God to live in and through him or her. That invitation is very often followed by an inner turning toward a transcendent peace, a profound change toward a life characterized by a more loving and spiritual perspective. What follows is a lifting of the spirit, a joy, and a new healed life.

Energy Work

Acupuncture

Acupuncture is an ancient Chinese therapy that involves the insertion of very thin needles into specific points on the body. These points are located along invisible lines known as meridians, each of which is believed to be linked to a different organ system. By stimulating these points, acupuncturists aim to unblock the flow of vital energy, called qi, and pronounced "chee," through the meridians and thus restore health to the body.

Although acupuncture does not provide an effective cancer treatment itself, it does help relieve cancer pain, chemotherapy-related nausea and vomiting, radiation-induced dry mouth, and post-treatment fatigue. I personally employ monthly acupuncture as part of my own wellness program.

If you are interested in understanding this modality and its potential application to your illness and treatment plan, visit http://acupuncturists.healthprofs.com/cam.

Hyperthermia

The term *hyperthermia* simply indicates a body temperature that is higher than normal. High body temperatures are often caused by illnesses, such as fever. But hyperthermia in cancer refers to heat treatment, the use of heat to destroy cancer cells.

Cells in the body exposed to higher than normal temperatures show marked inner-cellular changes. These changes may result in malignant cells becoming more likely to be affected by radiation therapy or chemotherapy. And very high temperatures can kill cancer cells outright. But high temperatures can injure or kill normal cells and tissues. This is why hyperthermia must be carefully controlled by someone with hyperthermia experience.

If you are interested in understanding this modality and its potential application to your illness and treatment plan, contact the Valley Cancer Institute in the Los Angeles, California, area (www.vci.org).

Shiatsu

Shiatsu is a form of acupressure that originated in Japan. It combines healing touch with a noninvasive acupuncture in order to help rebalance energy. It reduces stiffness, pain, fatigue, and stress, and it improves energy and sleep.

Therapeutic Touch/Reiki

Therapeutic touch or Reiki decreases stress and anxiety, helps reduce fatigue, aids in recovery from physical/emotional trauma, and helps minimize side effects of conventional cancer treatments.

Yoga

Gentle yoga is helpful for people dealing with illness, inviting them to listen and reconnect with their bodies. Through yoga you will gain a greater understanding of how you can support your body in healing. Start with hatha yoga, which focuses on simple and achievable movements, focused breathing exercises, and relaxation techniques. I personally like the DVD series *Yoga for Beginners*, which is widely available where books are sold.

If you are interested in understanding yoga and its potential application in your wellness quest, visit www.yogafinder.com.

BODYWORK

Alexander Technique

Decreases muscle strain, nerve pain, chronic pain, fatigue, and postsurgical weakness.

Chiropractic

Useful for musculoskeletal pain, particularly for the lower back. Decreases joint and muscle aches and releases tension. Improves range of motion. Increasing claims for improvements in general health and well-being.

Craniosacral

Head and neck massage. Treats muscle tension, injury, structural misalignment, and nerve dysfunction. Decreases stress.

Manual Lymph Drainage

Manual lymphatic drainage (MLD) is a safe, gentle massage technique that is used to treat many health conditions. It does not treat cancer itself but helps to improve symptoms of cancer treatments such as pain, neuropathy, lymphedema, scars, and postsurgical swelling.

Lymphedema is a condition that occurs in approximately 30 percent of cancer patients. It is a swelling that occurs most often in the arms or legs. Lymphedema is a result of an impaired lymphatic system due to chemotherapy, radiation, surgery, or removal of lymph nodes. It can be managed or prevented with the timely application of combined decongestive therapy (CDT). This involves (1) skin care, (2) exercise, (3) compression, and (4) manual lymph drainage.

If you are interested in understanding this modality and its potential application to your illness and treatment plan, visit www.klosetraining.com/TherapistDirectory.asp.

Massage

Massage is the systematic manipulation of soft tissues of the body to enhance health and healing and can be used to achieve an improved level of well-being. From a medical or therapeutic perspective, massage can help a person living with cancer by reducing pain, anxiety, and stress and providing caring touch.

Massaging the tumor itself is not recommended. However, people with cancer should not fear that massage is dangerous. In fact, massage can be a very important part of a complementary cancer care program.

There is no evidence to suggest that touch or gentle massage causes metastasis. But there is ample evidence that it greatly benefits many cancer patients, both physically and emotionally. In fact, touch addresses not only physical needs, but emotional, social, and spiritual needs as well.

Skilled touch can be beneficial at every stage of cancer treatment and recovery. Receiving comforting, attentive massage reminds us that the body can be a source of pleasure. It also can influence our ability to enjoy the present moment and feel our aliveness. A massage helps in reuniting body with heart, mind, and soul.

Excellent research has shown that massage can positively affect many cancer symptoms or side effects from conventional treatment regimens. These include nausea, fatigue, insomnia, and pain. Massage supports relaxation, which in turn supports immune function. As a result, thousands of cancer patients report an increased sense of well-being and a reduction in anxiety and muscle tension.

If you are interested in understanding more about massage and its potential application in your wellness quest, visit http://massagetherapists.healthprofs.com/cam.

Polarity Therapy

Emotional and physical energy balancing. Improves circulation. Relieves pain and stiffness. Increases energy, flexibility, and clarity.

Rolfing®

Deep muscle bodywork. Decreases stress, chronic pain, and stiffness. Improves breathing, mobility, energy, and posture.

GUIDE 4:
ALTERNATIVE CANCER THERAPIES

OVERVIEW

One of the reasons for my commitment to expand Cancer Recovery Foundation globally is to educate people to the fact that a wide variety of excellent anticancer therapies do exist, albeit not yet in Western medicine. This book is limited to helping people put in place an integrated cancer care program. Typically, that includes conventional medical care such as surgery, radiotherapy, chemotherapy, and/or hormone therapy.

Other treatments simply cannot be covered within the scope of this book. Yet they need exposure, too, especially for people who have had disappointment after disappointment with conventional medical options. What follows is a partial list of the alternative treatments that I know, firsthand, have effectively helped people with cancer extend life and improve quality of life. I offer this list without evaluation or endorsement. A simple Google search will yield information for your consideration.

Antineoplaston therapy	Chaparral
Hydrazine sulfate	Dr. Moerman's Anti-cancer diet
Hoxsey therapy	DMSO/hematoxylon therapy
Pau d'arco	Essiac
Wheatgrass therapy	Revici therapy
Chelation therapy	Mistletoe (Iscador)
Traditional Chinese medicine	Macrobiotics
Gaston Naessen's 714-X	Oxygen therapies
Immunoaugmentive therapy	Hyperthermia
Gerson therapy	Enderlein therapy

Three stand out as holding exceptional promise for wide-scale use. Antineoplastons seem especially promising for brain tumors. Iscador, widely used with much success in Germany, is plant-based and actually derived from mistletoe. Plus hyperthermia, or heat therapy. It is time, past time, that these three treatments are routinely integrated into conventional oncology care globally.

My aim here is to communicate to you a simple awareness that many other treatments exist. Many of these are superior to the conventional cancer treatments offered in North America and much of the world where Western medical practices are prominent.

AYURVEDA

Ayurveda is a holistic system of medicine from India. Its aim is to provide guidance regarding food and lifestyle so that healthy people can stay healthy and people with health challenges can improve their health.

Its recommendations will often be different for each person regarding which foods and which lifestyle they should follow. Ayurveda treatments are validated by observation, inquiry, direct examination, and knowledge derived from the ancient texts. The discipline believes that there are forces of energy that influence nature and human beings. These forces are called the Tridoshas. Because Ayurveda sees a strong connection between the mind and the body, much emphasis is placed on this aspect of health and healing.

If you are interested in understanding this modality and its potential application to your illness and treatment plan, visit www.yogaeverywhere.com/directory-ayurvedic.html.

HOMEOPATHY

Homeopathy administers prescriptive symptom-like medications, usually in low potencies. This triggers the body's own ability to combat illness and disease. Today, homeopathy is increasingly associated with fractionated dose chemotherapy where the physician monitors the results of a dilute-potency treatment before prescribing anything further. This results in minimizing side effects generally associated with cytotoxic drugs.

If you are interested in understanding this modality and its potential application to your illness and treatment plan, visit www.homeopathy.org/directory.html.

NATUROPATHIC MEDICINE

Naturopathic medicine is a part of healthcare emphasizing illness prevention, treatment, and the promotion of optimal health through the use of therapeutic methods and modalities that encourage the self-healing process. Naturopathic practice blends centuries-old knowledge of natural, non-toxic therapies with current advances in the understanding of health.

Naturopathic diagnosis and therapeutics incorporates both traditional approaches and, increasingly, therapies supported by scientific research drawn from peer-reviewed journals from many disciplines, including naturopathic medicine, conventional medicine, European complementary medicine, clinical nutrition, phytotherapy, pharmacognosy, homeopathy, psychology, and spirituality. Clinical research into natural therapies has become an increasingly important focus for naturopathic physicians.

Naturopathic medicine:

- Acknowledges the healing power of nature.
- Emphasizes disease prevention and encourages building health by assessing health risk factors and hereditary susceptibility to disease and making appropriate interventions to prevent illness.
- Identifies, treats, and removes the underlying causes of illness, rather than suppresses symptoms.
- Adheres to the dictum "First, do no harm." Utilizes methods and substances that minimize the risk of harmful side effects. Avoids, when possible, the harmful suppression of symptoms. Employs the least force necessary to diagnose and treat illness.
- Acknowledges the role of doctor as teacher to educate patients and encourage self-responsibility for health. Also honors the therapeutic value inherent in the doctor/patient relationship.
- Treats the whole person.

Naturopathic medical care can be utilized to help maintain the physical well-being of patients going through the various stages of cancer treatment. This includes both before and after chemotherapy, radiation, and surgery. Naturopathic medicine has been shown to alleviate the symptoms or negative side effects that often follow cancer treatment.

For patients who choose to explore targeted naturopathic cancer treatments, individualized programs are available. People who are in remission or cancer-free and would like to improve their overall health and well-being can also benefit from naturopathic medical approaches. Facilitating detoxification while supporting health and immune function is an important cornerstone in naturopathic cancer care.

A naturopath may also employ the therapeutic application of air, water, heat, cold, sound, light, and the physical modalities of electrotherapy, diathermy, ultrasound, hydrotherapy, hyperthermia, therapeutic exercise, and naturopathic manipulative therapy. This may be accomplished by specific therapies including:

- Intravenous vitamin C
- Intravenous glutathione
- Intravenous hydrogen peroxide
- Hyperthermia
- Chelation therapy
- Neural therapy
- Ozone therapy
- Colonics
- Constitutional hydrotherapy
- Hyperbaric oxygen therapy

In order to practice these specialized procedures, a naturopathic physician must undergo advanced training. Look especially for a Naturopathic Doctor (N.D.) with a degree from Bastyr University, the most-esteemed naturopathic medical school in the world.

If you are interested in understanding this approach to health and healing and its potential application to your illness and treatment plan, visit www.naturopaths.healthprofs.com/cam.

Traditional Chinese Medicine

Traditional Chinese medicine (TCM) practitioners use methods such as acupuncture, herbal formulas, diet and lifestyle counseling, and massage, as well as exercises such as tai chi and qigong to restore the flow of qi, vital energy, and the balance of yin and yang to the body.

TCM diagnosis is based on examination of the pulse and tongue as well as observation and extensive question asking. TCM views health as a state of harmony and balance between mind, body, and spirit.

Chinese medicine developed from tribal roots. By 200 BC, traditional Chinese medicine was firmly established. Even though they did not understand the body in the way that modern medicine does, ancient Chinese physicians recognized that the body provides sensitive signals about health and the nature of illness. These signals are perceived as symptoms such as abnormal temperature sensations, altered thirst, increases or decreases in appetite, and changes in emotional states.

A TCM examination is thorough and noninvasive. The practitioner will take a careful family and personal medical history, noting your body's reaction to stress and stimuli such as heat and cold. They will observe the color and form of your face and body, note the condition of your skin and nails, and look at your posture and even listen to the sound of your voice. The condition of your tongue, including its shape, color, and coating, also provides important data on the way your circulation and metabolism is affecting your internal organs. Your pulse will be felt at three different points on each wrist, each location corresponding, in TCM theory, to a different part of the body. Considered together, this information gives the practitioner a sense of your body's current functioning.

Acupuncture

We previously introduced acupuncture. It is a branch and central practice of traditional Chinese medicine. The key to understanding this acupuncture treatment is in the qi, the rivers of energy that flow through the body to nourish organs and tissues.

There are fourteen major acupuncture meridians, and each of these is believed to be associated with a particular part of the body. An obstruction or blockage in the movement of qi creates imbalance and pain in the body and can lead to disease.

By manipulating the acupuncture needles in a certain way, the practitioner attempts to bring energy to areas that are lacking or to create flow in areas that are blocked, bringing a sense of balance back to the body. Most people feel very relaxed during and after the treatment.

The National Institutes of Health Consensus Statement on Acupuncture concluded that *acupuncture has been found to be a promising treatment to help ease the side effects of conventional cancer therapies such as chemotherapy and radiation. It can also be effectively used to control pain, improve quality of life, and strengthen the immune system.*

TCM practitioners believe that in order for cancer to exist in the body, there must be certain factors and imbalances present to a greater or lesser degree. These factors include blood stagnation, energy weakness, phlegm, and environmental toxins.

Acupuncture is also used by TCM practitioners in an effort to counterbalance the damage actually caused by chemotherapy and radiation, thus helping the body to heal itself. TCM treatment may also help to support the immune system and digestive functioning.

In addition to acupuncture, a TCM practitioner may make recommendations on diet, exercise, herbs, and lifestyle modifications based on your current state of health and modify as needed.

If you are interested in understanding this modality and its potential application to your illness and treatment plan, visit www.tcmdirectory.com.

Guide 5:
Living Well

An important part of life after cancer is to be ever vigilant of the environments in which we live. With diet, exercise, and mind/body disciplines, we have now created an internal environment that maximizes our health and healing. But we also live in an external environment where factors such as sun exposure, chemical exposure, and even radio wave exposure have an unknown impact on our health.

Our lifestyle choices make a huge difference in our health and well-being. In this guide, I address two matters of environmental exposure that deeply concern me. First is cell phones, and second is chemicals in the home.

Cell Phones and Cancer

Q: Do cell phones cause cancer?
A: Maybe.

Q: Is there credible scientific evidence showing that radiation from a mobile phone has a biological impact?
A: Definitely.

Q: Should I be taking precautions in the use of my cell phone?

A: Absolutely.

"If cell phones were a type of food, they simply would not be licensed." This statement was not uttered by some uneducated anti-technology activist but rather was written by British physicist and two-time Nobel nominee Dr. Gerard Hyland. His statement was printed in the prestigious British medical journal the *Lancet*.

The safety of mobile phones is a subject few consumers ever think about. Just five years ago, the quality of the voice connection and longer battery life were the major concerns. That has changed.

Today the evidence is mounting that mobile telephony causes a range of adverse effects in people. The most significant research reveals concern about the possible connections between frequent cell phone use and neurological problems including an increased incidence of brain tumors. Other studies are also documenting higher rates of "head and neck cancers," which include mouth, nose, sinuses, salivary glands, throat, and lymph nodes in the neck.

In fact, there is growing evidence that mobile telephony, including cell phones and the myriad of new devices flooding the market, may be the greatest and most underestimated health threat in modern history. As a fellow cancer patient seeking to remain well, I want to know about such a threat and what I can do to minimize it.

Cellular Technology: 101

To gain a layman's understanding of this subject, a basic understanding of cell phone technology is necessary. Cell phones and cell phone towers emit radio-frequency energy. This energy is in the form of radio waves, microwaves actually, of what is called non-ionizing electromagnetic radiation. These invisible waves of energy move at the speed of light.

The basic transmission technology of mobile telephony is easily understood. A cell phone tower or base station antenna typically sends out microwaves at a rate of sixty watts. The actual handheld mobile device generates microwaves at rates between one and two watts. The antenna of a handset sends signals equally in all directions while a base station produces a beam that is much more directional, depending on line-of-sight connections with other cell phone towers and mobile devices in the area. It's like a giant spider web. It is also noteworthy to understand that the base stations themselves have lower-power side beams that are localized in the immediate vicinity of the tower.

The handheld device itself also emits a low-frequency electromagnetic field (EMF) associated with current from the phone's battery. With mobile devices that have an energy-saving discontinuous transmission mode, there is an even lower EMF, which occurs when the user is listening but not speaking.

There has been a significant shift in cell phone technology since cell phones came on the market. In the 1970s, the first big and bulky handheld devices relied on what is called analog signals. These radio waves were "on" all the time without interruption. Our understanding of analog signals showed they did little if any damage to living tissue except for a moderate increase in temperature.

The new technology, called "3G" and "4G," employs compressed digital signals using faster, smaller, and more powerful radio waves that are "pulsed" on and off rather than continuous. Because these devices are rapidly and repeatedly sending and receiving signals to the cell tower base stations, not just voice signals but the full range of multimedia services offered through today's mobile devices, the individual's cumulative exposure to pulsed microwave radiation can be much, much greater.

Cell Phone Biology: 101

Electromagnetic radiation is divided into two types: "ionizing" radiation such as found in X-rays and "non-ionizing" radiation found in cellular technology. There is clearly a biological impact to ionizing radiation such as from chest X-rays, radiation therapy used in many cancer treatments, and even the Transportation Security Administration's "backscatter" X-ray technology in use at many airports. Too much exposure and the risk of cancer dramatically increases.

Thermal Biological Risks

The use of cell phones also has a clear biological effect. The radio frequency energy produces heat. Think of a microwave oven as perhaps the best-known example. Exposure to radio frequency energy heats the body. And it is simple to record a warming of the body's temperature, especially at the point of contact with the cell phone. There is no question that exposing our heads to microwave energy as we talk on our cell phones results in a rise in temperature in the nearby tissue, a fact beyond dispute. In the world of cell phone safety, this "hot hypothesis" remains central to our understanding and concerns.

The amount of such heat produced in a living organism depends primarily on the intensity of the radiation, as well as the body's thermal self-regulation, once it has penetrated the tissue. Frighteningly, excellent research indicates that effects on health begin once the temperature rise exceeds only 1°C.

The central concern is the possibility this heating results in increasing numbers of brain tumors and head and neck cancers. But it is not only our head that is vulnerable. Among the most thermally sensitive areas of the body, because of their low blood supply, are the eyes and the testes. Cataract formation and reduced sperm counts are well documented in studies of acute exposure to microwave energy.

Although much of the evidence on the link between cell phone use and cancer is disputed by the National Cancer Institute (U.S.), research from the World Health Organization's (WHO) International Agency for Research on Cancer as well as the European Environmental Agency is unequivocal. Their position is that the evidence is significant and growing showing microwave radiation employed in cell phone technology, and the resulting "hot spots" it creates, is linked to higher cancer incidence.

In an exhaustive review released in 2011 by WHO, it was documented that people who have used cell phones for half an hour a day for more than a decade have about twice the risk of glioma, a rare kind of brain tumor. Not surprisingly, the glioma appeared most often on the side of their head where these people hold their phone.

Brain cancers typically take decades to develop. The fact that such tumors are being found after ten years in cell phone users with relatively light exposure by today's usage standards is sobering.

Non-Thermal Biological Risks

Could it be possible that pulsed microwave radiation used in cell phone technology also exerts non-thermal influences on the human body? It seems so.

This issue centers on the frequency or oscillations of the microwaves and their impact on physiological processes as fundamental as cell division. Just to be clear, when we speak here of the "frequency," this has to do with the characteristics of the vibrations of the radio waves. This is independent from the heating of tissue and does not refer to how "frequently" we are exposed to these.

Microwave radiation has certain well-defined frequencies, some of which emulate the human body's biological electrical activities. Thus the incoming radio wave can potentially interfere with the orderly and exquisitely balanced functions of the body. It's analogous to reception distortions on a car radio.

Although this non-thermal cell biology frequency premise is not without its vocal skeptics, there is growing experimental evidence to support it. At the cellular level, the observed evidence of exposure to microwave radiation includes:

- A "switch on" of certain cell division process
- Reduced lymphocyte toxicity

- Increased membrane permeability
- Increases in chromosome aberrations

In animal studies, non-thermal microwave radiation exposure influences include:

- Depression of immune function in chickens
- Increase in chick embryo mortality
- Increased permeability of blood-brain barrier in laboratory mice
- Changes in brain chemistry, including dopamine levels, in laboratory mice
- Increases in DNA strand breaks in laboratory mice
- Increases in lymphoma in mice

In human studies, non-thermal microwave radiation exposures, and similarly conditioned exposures, include demonstrations of:

- Headache
- Blood pressure changes
- Sleep disorders with shortening of rapid-eye-movement periods

Non-thermal effects of cell phone radiation have proved to be quite controversial in the scientific community. The health problems are reported anecdotally and formal confirmation of such reports, based on epidemiological studies, are still to be completed. But to deny this possibility yet admit the importance of banning the use of mobile phones on airplanes and in hospitals, both prohibitions driven solely by concerns about non-thermal interference, is grossly inconsistent.

We have underplayed the threat of cell phone radiation too long. The message has been slow to capture public attention. Even government acknowledgment of the problem is minimal. And because much of the research into the potential dangers of cell phones has been funded by the cell phone industry, negative findings are routinely dismissed. It's understandable, as such information would be detrimental to cell phone sales.

It is not surprising that author Devra Davis points out in her excellent book *Disconnect*, "There has not been a lot of truly independent research in this field." In one of the most enlightening passages, Davis chronicles the work of Dariusz Leszczynski from Finland. He holds two doctoral degrees and is a research professor in Finland's National Radiation and Nuclear Safety Authority. He has served as a visiting professor at Harvard Medical School and is currently an adjunct professor of bioelectro-magnetics at a medical school in Hangzhou, China. Impressive credentials.

In 2002, Leszczynski's research showed that after just one hour of exposure to pulsed cell phone signals, the same signals that are in the phones millions of people use each and every day, changes were recorded in the shape and character of endothelial cells, the tiny membranes that line our blood vessels. The reason this is so critically important is that breakdowns in endothelial cells are thought to be direct precursors to the formation of malignant cells. In short, his work showed that even low levels of microwave radiation may impact the formation of cancer, especially brain cancers.

What's more, collaborative research showed children are more vulnerable to radiation than adults. It makes perfect sense. Radiation that penetrates only two inches into the brain of an adult will reach much deeper into the brain of a child. Their young skulls are thinner and their brains contain more fluid that absorbs the heat. Even though we know this, we allow children, and especially young adolescents, to freely use this technology. In fact, many of the new "applications" for mobile technology are aimed squarely at this age group.

Such findings should have had a dramatic effect on the cell phone industry and cell phone safety. They did not.

Professor Leszczynski was asked about his groundbreaking study during a visit to Washington, D.C., in 2010 where he testified before the U.S. Senate. He said, ". . . we clearly showed that radiation from a cell phone had a biological impact. [Now] the world can no longer pretend that the only problems with cell phones occur after you can measure a change in temperature."

But we do keep pretending . . . all of us, including governments, research scientists, the cell phone industry, and especially cell phone consumers. Most people are totally unaware that radio frequency radiation causes biological changes to their body. Or if they are among the few who are aware, most are in denial regarding the seriousness of the problem.

Protecting Yourself and Your Loved Ones

We can do better. Below is a list of personal actions you can implement right now. Do so and you will be doing all possible to keep you and your family safe from cell phone radiation.

- Switch to a low-radiation phone. Consider replacing your phone with one that emits the lowest radiation possible and still meets your needs.
- Use a headset or speaker. Headsets emit much less radiation than handsets. Choose either wired or wireless. Unfortunately, experts are split on which version is safer. Some wireless headsets emit continuous, low-level radiation, so take yours off your ear when you're not on a call. Using your phone in speaker mode also reduces radiation to the head.
- Listen more and talk less. Your phone emits radiation when you talk or text, but not when you're receiving messages. Listening more and talking less reduces your exposures.
- Hold the phone away from your body. Holding the phone away from your torso when you're talking on your headset or speaker—rather than against your ear, in a pocket, or on your belt—means your soft body tissues absorb less radiation.
- Text rather than talk. Mobile phones use less power and radiation to send text than voice. And unlike when you speak with the phone at your ear, texting keeps radiation away from your head.
- If you have a poor signal, stay off the phone. Fewer signal

bars on your phone means that it emits more radiation to get the signal to the tower. Make and take calls when your phone has a strong signal.

- Limit children's cell phone use. A child's brain absorbs twice the cell phone radiation as an adult's. Health agencies in at least a dozen countries recommend limits for children's cell phone use, such as for emergency situations only.
- Skip the radiation shield. Radiation shields such as antenna caps or keypad covers reduce the connection quality and force the phone to transmit at a higher power with higher radiation.
- Store your cell phone in a backpack or purse. If you must carry it mounted on your belt, turn the keypad to face your body because the antenna is on the back and it emits much more radiation compared to the keyboard.
- Don't sleep with your cell phone on a table next to the bed or under your pillow.
- Pregnant women should keep the phones away from their abdomen.
- Use your cell phone less. High-frequency users have higher incidence of reported neurological disease. Use a landline whenever it is available.

A Personal Appeal

In the end, I certainly am not advocating banning the use of cell phones. I use mine safely every day of the week. But I am urging cell phone manufacturers to make their products safer. Safer technology exists; it is past time to implement it. Plus, I am asking for each of us to be fully aware of the dangers and take personal responsibility for curbing our exposure, and our family's exposure, to cell phone radiation. It's the only way to be certain we are not damaging our bodies every time we are on the phone.

OTHER ENVIRONMENTAL THREATS

Cell phones are just the tip of the iceberg. We live in a sea of chemicals, a world of environmental unknowns. I am convinced that exposure to environmental contaminants has a stronger impact on cancer risk than previously believed. That is virtually the only way cancers with non-genetic links can be explained.

That belief is backed by a recent report from the President's Cancer Panel. Despite a growing body of evidence linking environmental exposures to cancer in recent years, the panel noted that it was "particularly concerned to find that the true burden of environmentally induced cancer has been grossly underestimated."

The report, entitled "Reducing Environmental Cancer Risk: What We Can Do Now," pointed out that although there are nearly 80,000 chemicals currently on the market in the United States, only about 200 of them have been studied for their impact on the human body. Many other chemicals are understudied and most are largely unregulated. Exposure to potential environmental carcinogens is widespread, and the National Cancer Program has not adequately addressed the "grievous harm" from this group of carcinogens, the President's Cancer Panel concludes.

"There remains a great deal to be done to identify the many existing but unrecognized environmental carcinogens and to eliminate those that are known from our daily lives—our workplaces, schools, and homes," said panel chair LaSalle D. Leffall, Jr., M.D., Professor of Surgery at Howard University College of Medicine in Washington, D.C.

"The increasing number of known or suspected environmental carcinogens compels us to action, even though we may currently lack irrefutable proof of harm," he said in a statement.

The panel advised President Obama "... to use the power of your office to remove the carcinogens and other toxins from our food, water, and air that needlessly increase healthcare costs, cripple our nation's productivity, and devastate American lives." Sadly, the nation's largest cancer organization, the American Cancer Society, dismissed the conclusions of the report.

Most worrisome is the accumulation of certain synthetic chemicals in humans and in the food chain. Possible combination effects of low doses of multiple chemicals, potential radiation risks from medical imaging devices, and the large number of industrial chemicals that have not been adequately tested lead to a worrisome situation. Of course, the potentially greater susceptibility of children is a matter of prime importance. But laws to regulate and test this industry have been virtually nonexistent.

This is a long-running debate. But the dilemma is that there literally have been thousands of new chemicals coming into the marketplace, and we have limited knowledge of their toxicity. Because many of these agents have not been screened, it is not known what health effect, if any, exposure to these chemicals will have.

The President's Cancer Panel reported that the "prevailing regulatory approach in the United States is reactionary rather than precautionary," meaning that human harm must be proven before action is taken to remove or reduce exposure to an environmental toxin. This approach should be reversed, and replaced with a precautionary prevention-oriented strategy, according to the report.

The President's Cancer Panel was established by the National Cancer Act of 1971, and is charged with monitoring the National Cancer Program and reporting annually to the president. Between September 2008 and January 2009, the panel held four meetings to evaluate the state of environmental cancer research, policy, and programs addressing the known and potential effects of environmental exposures on cancer. They received testimony from forty-five invited experts from academia, government, industry, the environmental and cancer advocacy communities, and the public.

The panel recommended concrete actions that government, industry, and individuals can take to reduce cancer risk related to environmental contaminants, excess radiation, and other harmful exposures. The recommendations for individuals include filtering tap water and eating organic foods.

Additional key recommendations include:

- Increase, broaden, and improve research regarding environmental contaminants and human health.
- Raise consumer awareness of environmental cancer risks and improve understanding and reporting of known exposures.
- Raise healthcare provider awareness of environmental cancer risks and the effects of exposure.
- Enhance efforts to eliminate unnecessary radiation-emitting medical tests and to ensure that radiation doses are as low as reasonably achievable without sacrificing quality.
- Aggressively address the toxic environmental exposures the American military has caused, and to improve response to associated health problems among both military personnel and civilians.

To date, one specific focus has been on bisphenol A (BPA), which is widely used in the production of polycarbonate plastics and epoxy resins. It is found in plastic food and drink containers. In its report, the panel noted that over the past decade, more than 130 studies have linked the chemical to breast cancer, obesity, and other disorders.

The nation's first ban on BPA was passed in Suffolk County, New York. It eliminated the use of the chemical in children's products. Several states, including Washington, Maryland, Wisconsin, Minnesota, and Connecticut, have recently banned BPA from baby bottles and other children's food and beverage containers. California, Vermont, New York, and Illinois have similar legislation pending.

Outside of the United States, Canada has prohibited the use of BPA in baby products. Denmark has banned its use in any food containers for young children. The French senate has also backed a proposal to ban its use in baby bottles.

The U.S. Food and Drug Administration (FDA) reviewed the safety of BPA in three separate sessions. In the last review it reversed its previous position, stating that it now has "some concern about the potential effects of BPA on the brain, behavior, and in fetuses, infants, and young children."

As the public debate rages, I suggest you and I take more direct and immediate action. Here are ten simple and practical things to do that help limit your exposure to environmental toxins right in your home and in your daily life.

ENVIRONMENTAL TOXINS TOP 10 CHECKLIST

1. Take off your shoes. Leave your shoes at the door so you do not carry outside chemicals into the home.
2. Use "green" cleaning supplies. Choose toxic-free cleaners. Leave your family living and breathing healthier.
3. Choose "safe" laundry products. Avoid detergents that contain phthalates, dyes, perfumes, and chlorine bleach. These dangerous chemicals in your laundry can be absorbed into your family's skin and lungs.
4. Test for radon. Radon is a naturally occurring gas, but it is dangerous when found in homes and is the second leading cause of lung cancer. This odorless gas can go undetected without testing.
5. Know your plastics. Learn what plastics are safe for eating and drinking. Do not microwave food in any plastic container, even those that state they are "microwave safe." Do not cover foods to be microwaved with plastic wrap. Leeched chemicals and dangerous toxins are released in the heating process.
6. Test your water. Many families unknowingly have dangerous chemicals in their water. Private systems should be tested yearly.
7. Know your foods. Purchase certified organic foods whenever possible.
8. Rethink your lawn care. Avoid using dangerous pesticides and insecticides on your lawn. Both contain cancer-causing chemicals that remain in the lawn for weeks and to which children are easily exposed.

9. Air out attached garages. Park outside when possible. Leave garage doors open to air out fumes for at least ten minutes after parking your car. Install a garage ventilation system.
10. Choose toxic-free paints and building supplies. Purchase toxic-free materials when building, remodeling, or doing home-improvement projects. This will limit the amount of toxic chemicals that linger in your home.

Environmental factors are the next major area of inquiry in the world of cancer. The next ten years will see major changes in public policy on these matters. Don't wait. Act now. You will benefit with greater health and well-being.

My Cancer Recovery Contract

I hereby devote the next year of my life to "Creating Wellness."
In addition to my chosen treatment, I commit my full intent
and focused efforts to getting well again.

I will:

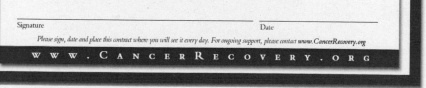

Medical:
- Continually research and understand all my treatment options;
- Implement a treatment plan that has my highest confidence; and
- Monitor the results both personally and with my healthcare team.

Nutrition:
- Consume a plant-based whole food diet;
- Eliminate refined "whites;" add bountiful fresh "colors;" and
- Implement a vitamin/mineral/herbal supplement program.

Exercise:
- Discover a physical activity that is "fun;"
- Commit to daily "fun;" and
- As a result, capture the emotion of joy.

Attitude:
- Become an expert on the mind/body connection;
- Focus my mind on healing, not on the problems of treatment; and
- Constantly affirm my health improvement.

Support:
- Nurture relationships that uplift;
- Put toxic relationships "on hold;" and
- Bond with others who are deeply committed to survivorship.

Spiritual:
- Live in constant connection with God.
- Release, let go and forgive all hostility in my life;
- Embrace gratitude as my way of life; and
- Practice unconditional love in thought, word and deed.

I hereby commit to traveling this incredible path to living well. And I affirm,

"I am cancer-free, a picture of health! Thank you, God!"

Signature   Date

Please sign, date and place this contract where you will see it every day. For ongoing support, please contact www.CancerRecovery.org